ENGINEERING MEDICAL MIRACLES

Return to Health Using Today's Technology

Dr. Thomas A. Santucci, DC, CNS

This book is written for
my wife, my children,
and my extended family
with the hope
that they will inherit or create
a more sophisticated and ethical medical reality.

To the many patients
that have provided
such a deep sense of wonder,
I would like to express
my deep appreciation for their
spirit, tenacity and bravery.

Acknowledgements

I do much of my writing when I am on the road attending Functional Medicine and Neurology seminars. In this place, my brain is flush with fresh ideas and seeded with the gems of some truly remarkable thinkers. These people never fail to impress the practitioner in me with their reasoned, researched, impassioned advancement of our kind of medicine.

Jeff Bland - who I think started it all. He taught us to that is was possible to achieve "Normal Miracles" in Patient Centric Care Dr. Fredrick Carrick - a true and appropriately eccentric genius in a Chiropractor's body. Dr. Andy Barlow - who may be the smartest man in Mississippi and who gave me the technical Neurology to achieve everyday miracles. Dr Le for demonstrating that shades of grey may be as important than the facts I know. Dr Peter Santucci (my dad) for persistently displaying the standards of excellence.

Forward

Integrative *Functional Medicine* offers a real life opportunity to correct the course of healthcare. Rational, research-based protocols that address the cause of the complex health problems in a patient oriented model.

Now these **everyday miracles** are establishing a new standard of practice for the discerning patient and enlightened practitioner.

I have felt for some time that it is necessary to chronicle the evolution of **Neurometabolic** Functional Medicine so that the lessons, methods and important safeguards we have so painstakingly derived are not lost in the excitement and chaos of new discoveries or obscured by the sub-specialties.

New to the Medical field, Functional testing and protocols were initially disregarded by the Neurologists, Endocrinologists and Internal Medicine docs because of "unwarranted" claims to correct "incurable" conditions. This is changing.

Much of the perspective of this book stems from my background as the son of Medical Parents, Georgetown educated, who enjoyed an intense Washington DC and Silicon Valley Business career prior to becoming a doctor at age 40.

I was classically trained as a Chiropractor. My medical education started with the Orthopedic and holistic orientation of that profession, progressed to the biochemistry of Functional Medicine and has ended with the brain-oriented work of Functional Neurology and qEEG Neurofeedback.

Each of these sub-specialties employs a way of thinking and an intrinsic belief system that becomes a kind of creed that it's practioners follow. This is perhaps justified by their substantial advances and very real tangible clinical results, **but also limits them**.

In each case, I have felt strongly that it was necessary to avoid "drinking the cool aid" of any one sub specialty.

Clinically, the apparently simple solution has never yielded good results for the support of Complex Conditions. In the early days of trying to understand Fatigue and Pain Syndromes, we needed to develop solutions that combined inputs from the vastly different worlds of neurology and biochemistry.

Recently, this work has progressed into a potent mix of machines and processes, integrating sophisticated Neurofeedback equipment and PEMF generators in an effort to effectively support cognitive conditions like depression, anxiety and memory loss.

The goal of the book is not so much to provide specific tactics, but rather the broad strokes to **recover and sustain your health** with 50 years of Functional Medicine insights.

The contributions of many *Neurometabolic* **solutions** are covered. Interventions and concepts are meant to be presented in a straightforward and understandable manner.

It is my hope that *Neurometabolic*[1] changes will provide a stage for the **next phase of health interventions** that hold the promise of significantly increasing vitality and extending life.

---

[1] I am distinguishing Functional Medicine from a brand of Integrative Medicine "Medipractors" where practitioners substitute natural biochemical solutions for protocols which mimic the old pharmacological ones.

PART 1

Introduction

ORGANIZATION OF THIS BOOK

FUNCTIONAL MEDICINE FOR IDIOTS
MY WORKING THEORIES

This is really 3 Books. (Sorry!) I have tried to be true to the etiology of some of the important stepping stones in the progression of functional medicine.

I **The first section attempts to offer some *context* of** the problems patients encountered with the business medicine model of the last 50 years and maps out the fundamentals of the ***Functional Medicine*** response.

II **The second section introduces *Functional Medicine Protocols*** and methods for addressing health concerns. I have taken about two times as much space in this book in this area as I intended.

III **The third section describes the onset of *Functional Neurology*** in the 1990's with its improved diagnostics and ability to address the "incurable" neurological illnesses.

IV **Lastly, the impact of the new *Computer and Energy therapies*** is introduced.

My Working Theories

You cannot "do medicine" without some kind of working belief system. These are some observations and basic assumptions of my practice and against which this book is written.

Sort of a "Functional Medicine for Idiots" Section

1. The first rule is that **"Everything Counts"**. When dealing with our organ systems, you can't leave anything out. You need to evaluate all of the different systems- digestion, liver detoxification, cardiovascular performance, neurology, immunity and emotions. This is the first contribution of **Functional Medicine**.

For example, when dealing with energy, you can't eat poorly, metabolize inefficiently, detoxify incompletely or ignore the composition and quality of food if you want the energy system to work well for very long. This particular point has become such a key issue that Food is now considered **"upstream medicine"**, a vital component of our very existence on this earth.

Understanding "what to worry about" and "what is less important" is a key skill in modern health management. Example: The distinction of Wheat versus Rice in your diet is probably important. White rice versus Brown rice arguably isn't.

2. **The bad stuff in the news actually impacts your life.** Our toxic world is beginning to have a **poisonous effect on our health**. Everything from the GMO grains to global warming affects us in some way. This now includes plastics, Styrofoam, industrial metals, food antigens, as well as, toxic energy from cell phones, solar radiation and microwaves, all of which are increasingly adding toxins to our experience.

3. There is a huge delay in the introduction of **Medical research** in the United States. For many reasons it has become **difficult for the medical community to quickly embrace new methods** of care even though they are well documented in research. In the face of abysmal performance in cardiovascular and cancer interventions, we still cling to **50-year-old notions** and their pharmaceutical solutions. **Statins, chemotherapy, and other harsh pharmaceuticals still pervade our medical landscape when the current literature offers far more hopeful solutions**

4. **"Fix the Problem where it is."**
Health can be divided into physical, biochemical, neural and energetic realities or States. Analyzing and correcting a problem in its appropriate state is the most direct and usually the most effective solution. That means treating physical problems at the muscle, joint and nerve level (not with drugs). That means treating neurological imbalances with Neurofeedback or rehab (not with drugs). That means treating biochemical imbalances with food (not drugs).

> *Health exists in multiple states – Physical, Biochemical, Neurological & Energetic. It is almost always more effective to correct a problem in the state of health from which it originated.*
>
> *T. Santucci*

5. **Quantum physics** with its elegant notions of life as a giant interrelated **energetic field** has begun to replace Newtonian (matter is solid) understandings just as Wikipedia and the internet have replaced the Merriam Webster Dictionary and the encyclopedia. **Quantum physics brings the reality that there is more space and more energy in the spaces between matter than in the matter itself. We are made out of less than 1% matter and over 99% energy!**

This means, that being a realist in medicine includes the understanding and application of energy.

6. **Technology is changing the existing doctor to doctor relationships in Medicine**. Most new breakthroughs combine existing specialties. Functional medicine practitioners broke down these barriers by holding themselves responsible for a cross section of organ systems. The reason that the Endocrinologist is likely to miss a Thyroid remediation is that **he is trained to disregard** the causes of the autoimmune attack in hypothyroidism. He only knows that it is a **destructive autoimmune disease** and tries to quell the symptoms using hormone replacement. A broader approach would look to the existence of the **other** autoimmune diseases which are likely caused by this patient's triggers in combinations with that individual's immune and DNA expression.

This is the source of significant controversy because the introduction of newer methods does not allow the restrictive safe harbors of specialization in which medicine is currently organized.

7. **Some of the best Solutions contain doctor and** patient initiatives. *The day of medicine-led health revolutions is past.* There is a popular statement in alternative medical circles that Polio was the last great medical victory **and that was in 1952!**

The remainder of the significance advances in public health performance have been from hygiene and nutritional improvements in the habits of everyday people.

In reality - there is a powerful potential in having a coordinated mix of practitioner directed advances and patient-managed initiatives. This means adding common sense, current research and scientific breakthroughs to medical and support protocols.

Introduction - To the optimistic and uninitiated, the accounting of the difficulties of Western Medical performance seems bizarre.It did to me.

Our performance shortfalls in infant mortality, drug use, obesity, lifespan and stress levels are all researched and documented in the literature.

It is not my intention to be the herald of these details, but rather to understand them and incorporate them into the landscape of the creation of a modern medical practice.

For those who need more, I would direct the reader to the many brave accounts of the authors who have formally researched these issues. (See works by Jeff Bland, Mark Hyman, the Functional Medicine Institute, etc. or as current as Meghan O'Rourke's article in the Atlantic)

It seems like the American health care system had its *own* health crisis. This has created a default position to very low level health care and has an opportunity to rebuild into a much better thing. This is the story of some of the inroads into that rebuilding.

Much of this work is born out of perspectives originating in **Functional Medicine and later Functional Neurology.** Recently new energetic and **Quantum level healing** have added a level of intervention that is making non-drug and non-surgical choices the sensible and effective alternative.

I have organized this section into a series of Statements that taken together show a medical "playing field" that hamstrings doctors, squashes innovation, limits important research and maintains archaic standards of practice.

PART II

What is going on in healthcare?

BACKGROUND ON THE
MEDICAL ENTERPRISE

THE EFFECTS OF ENVIRONMENT
THE DISEASES OF MODERN MAN

U.S. Health Care

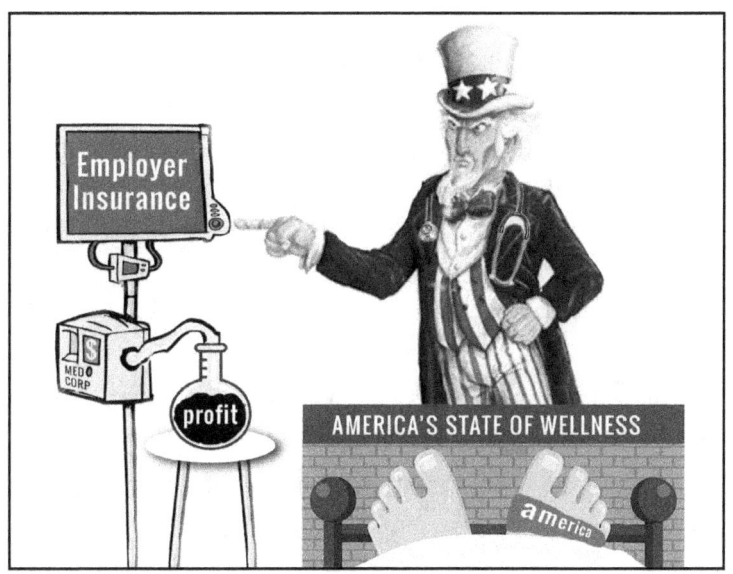

While employing bigger budgets and having more doctors and more specialists in the US than any other country, we somehow manage to have one of **the worst performing medical systems on the planet**.[2]

---

[2]   US health care: A reality check on cross-country comparisons H.E. Frech, Stephen T. Parente, John Hoff July 11, 2012

Doctors do not have time to do it right

In the last 30 years, the prevailing model for Doctor – Patient Interface has been radically modified.

> *The General Practitioner is given an average of 8 minutes to correctly assess and remediate an ever more complex set of medical conditions.*

All too often, specialists are increasingly satisfied with providing "**Standard of Care**"[3] treatment that have not proven effective against the rising tide of neurologic and autoimmune diseases.

Care standards protect the practitioner but severly limit diagnostic and treatment options. This has trapped doctors and patients into a loosing strategy.

---

[3] Tuesday, March 18, 2014 The "Standard of Care" Posted by William Paolo *A guest post by William Paolo (@paolomd1), the Program Director of Emergency Medicine at SUNY Upstate*.

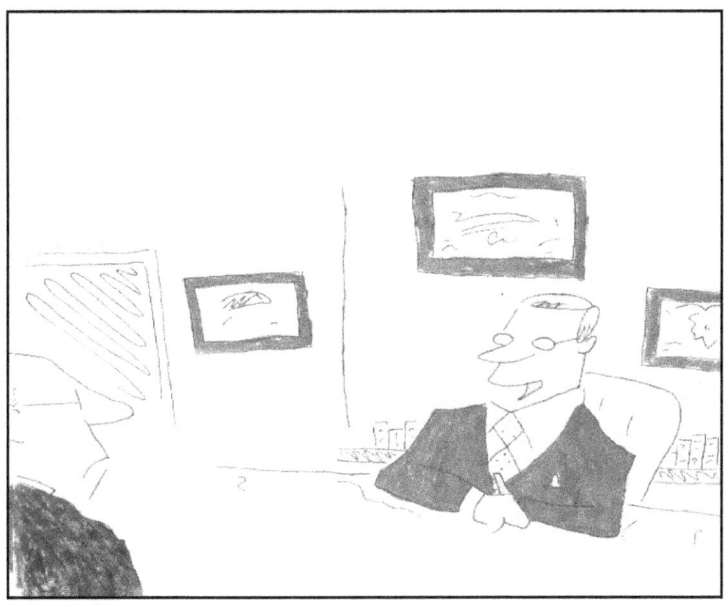

*Try to focus less on a cure and more on
a treatment that fits your budget*

Medical Research
is compromised

The next problem encountered in the administration of a healthy US Health Care system is the method in which **medical research** is utilized. Medical research was regularly manipulated in the last century. Multiple clinical trials were started and the ones that agreed with the manufacturer were published. This got so bad that Congress mandated new rules for publishing medical trials and remains a very real concern in the "healthy skepticism" crowd.

Most Practitioners are not Innovators

Evidence-based does not necessarily mean "Current". The late adoption of "proven research" by many doctors permeates Medicine.

Doing things "the way we used to do them" is disastrous in a field where the body of knowledge doubles every 3 to 5 years. Maloney's chart helps explains the phenomenon of early adapters to the general acceptance of an idea.

Part of the framework of the Adoption Curve is the behavior toward medical breakthroughs. New technologies that may threaten the "standard of care" are often harassed and downplayed. With media and Medical associations at their side, many doctors cling to decades old protocols.

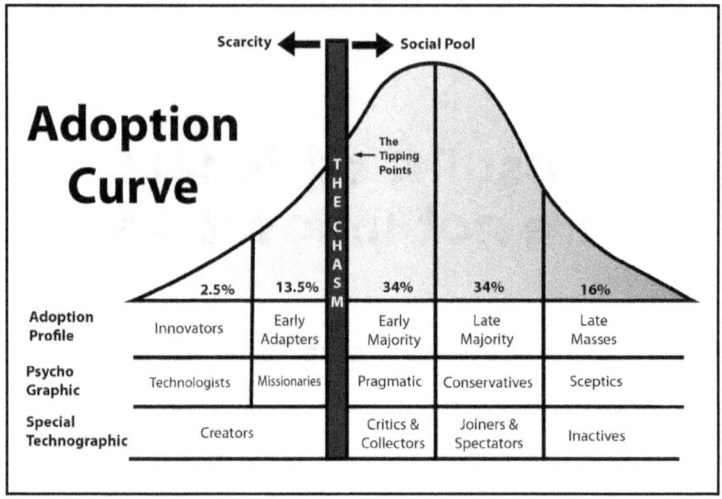

- Initially new changes are labeled as unreasonable or silly or preposterous.

- Next it is seen as unfounded in literature or even dangerous.

- After enough anecdotal evidence is amassed, then the new product or procedure is viewed as something "that might work on some people".

- In the next phase, there is the beginning of acceptance and the late adopters usually attempt to regulate the innovation. Saying that "This is so good or powerful or important that it needs to be managed by us".

This ploy has been repeated with supplements, nutraceuticals, metal chelators and IV vitamin therapy. Thee have all traveled from designations of "inappropriate and unsafe" to "so important that they need to be managed by a Medical Doctor."

Healthcare's early adopters innovate with techniques & methods and Medicine's late adopters ask for **Research**. This seemingly innocuous requirement for research is often **a smoke screen to maintain position or profit.**

Drug Companies Significantly Influence or Own Parts of Health Care

Research is largely financed by pharmaceutical companies and that published results with "gold standard, placebo-controlled, double blind structures" often favor drug and surgical options.

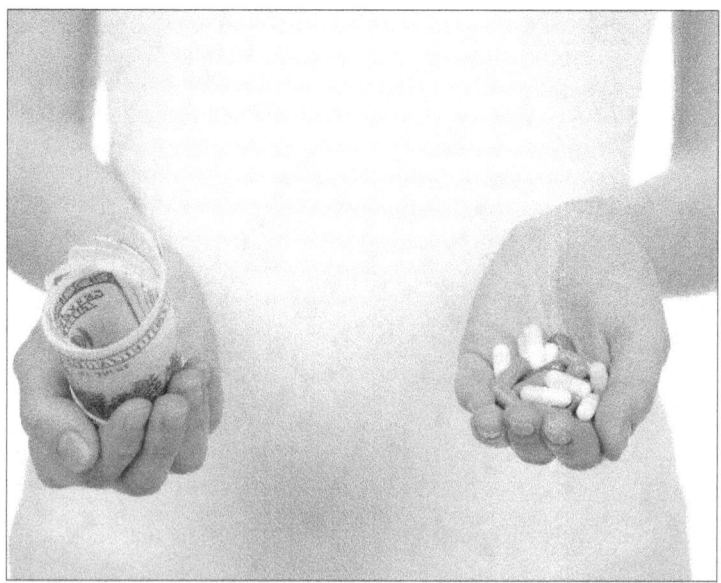

Due to the extraordinary costs, most medical research is tilted toward well-funded drug companies. Pharmaceutical-based models have been oversold by drug companies virtually ensuring that **medications** are the recommended form of support. The effect is that the United Stated uses **400% more meds** than any other developed nation.[4]

---

[4] CHART OF THE DAY: Americans Will Continue To Spend More On Drugs Than The Rest Of The World In 2016 Lisa MahapatraRead more: http://www.businessinsider.com/us-spending-more-on-pharmaceuticals-2013-1#ixzz35E3MtpWt

Insurance Companies Determine a Large Part of Medical Protocols

The last of the big snags with the US HealthCare System is that **Insurance Companies** are the day to day arbitrators of standards of care. By limiting medical payouts, Insurance companies have become the enforcers of compromised medicine.

> *A doctor that wishes to provide a level of service that doesn't match the "standard of care protocol" is essentially on their own – They are exposed medically, legally, financially and socially.*

Patients are not happy with the Conventional Medical Status quo

It seems that doctors are no longer controlling medicine. Patients and doctors have been trapped by a failed paradigm. Not surprising, this style of perfunctory and drug-based care has been widely criticized for its poor diagnostic and clinical performance.

Twenty years ago this would not have mattered. But in the internet age, where information is power and the consumer has a collective voice, awareness of sophisticated modalities is driving a patient fueled revolution. *It is here where hope lies.*

Where Are We Now?

The Diseases of Modern Man

The new set of challenges to our health are taking the form of ever more complex conditions that **do not confine themselves to one body system or one type of medicine.**

Chronic Fatigue Syndrome, Peripheral Neuropathy, Fibromyalgia, Thyroid Disease, Alzheimer's, Dementias, Celiac Disease and Autistic Spectrum conditions routinely go unresolved in this country.

Across the board, US progress on major health initiatives have essentially been fruitless. **The national statistics are no better today for** resolution of Diabetes, Cancer or Cardiac patients than they were **50 years ago.**[5] Diabetes, in particular is on the rise.

---

[5] NCHS Data Brief, Number 88, March 2012
75 Years of Mortality in the United States, 1935–2010

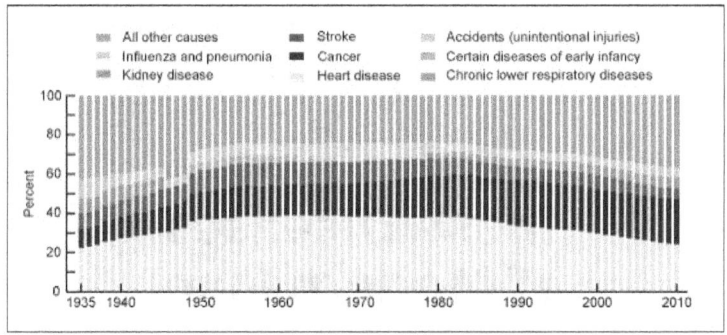

*Death from Serious Illnesses has not
decreased in over 50 years*

Instead of revolutionizing medicine, some of the new technology has just made it more *expensive*. See the technology section in Part III of this book to find technology that *is* working.

Why do we care? No other set of conditions has highlighted the shortfalls of specialist-based, standard of practice medicine like the "Diseases of Modern Man".

Explaining these Diseases of Modern Man

The combination of food antigens, toxins from the environment and stress are responsible for many of the Diseases of Modern Man and the significant rise of autoimmune diseases we are now facing in America.

Because ignorance, denial and minimalism pervade the conventional thinking on toxins, I think it is useful to provide some details on where some of sources of poisons and autoimmune triggers in our country.

Environmental toxins

In the San Francisco Bay, **one can readily be exposed to heavy metals in the form of arsenic, lead and mercury from the bay, dioxin and bha-bht in the food and petroleum and chemical additives from pumping your own gasoline.**[6]

Tissue biopsies regularly turn up Styrene (a form of Styrofoam) in our tissues. The EPA National Human Adipose Tissue Survey for 1986 identified **Styrene** in 100% of all samples of human fat tissue taken in 1982 in the US. From the perspective of the past - It seems like an improbable or inflated list of environmental risks. Unfortunately, it is the situation that we have inherited for ourselves and our families.

In 100 years, we have acutely raised the global toxicity levels by an estimated 40% affecting all of the world's air and all of the world's oceans.

---

[6]   Our Poisoned Bay / Despite end to direct piping of sewage, pollution worse now than 30 years ago
Glen Martin, Chronicle Staff Writer
Published 4:00 am, Monday, August 2, 1999

Nothing in human evolution can keep up with the detoxification and molecular reclassification necessary to endure these levels of toxins.

Toxic chemicals and stress have become the metabolic originator and fuel for unrelenting Cancer, Heart Disease and Autoimmune Diseases.

Stress
(Think Inflammation)

We now know that lifestyle stress can be as dangerous to our systems as trauma. The introductions of **cortical hormones increase our blood pressure, interferes with digestion and sleep and lowers our immune response.**[7] Stress is a major contributor to heart disease, blood sugar dysregulation and poor cognitive performance. It becomes another common, but still toxic trigger of the diseases of modern man.

The causes of stress are everywhere. Work, money and the economy are the most common causes of our stress. After that, we worry about relationships, responsibilities and health, with jobs, housing and personal safety to a slightly lesser extent.

---

[7] American Pyschological Association

Causes of Stress and Physical Symptoms

What Goes Wrong		How We React	
Money	75%	Irritability or Anger	42%
Work	70%	Anxiety	39%
Economy	67%	Fatigue	37%
Relationships	56%	Depression	37%
Family	53%	Lack of Energy	35%
Health	53%	Headache	32%
Job	49%	Feeling Like Crying	30%
House Cost	49%	Upset Stomach	24%
Safety	32%	Tension	24%

We generally **react to stress** with anger and anxiety which can turn into depression and fatigue over time. This conversion depends on the level of reserves we maintain to combat the stressors.

Stress acts as an important contributor to cellular inflammation and as such is a key component of the Neurometabolic diseases of modern man.

Our Troubled Antigens – the autoimmune epidemic

The last and most insidious precondition for Chronic Illness is Autoimmune Activity. Our immune systems are designed to make a decision on every molecule we come in contact with as to whether we **accept it as part of our genetic potential or reject it as an invader.**

This system is now so completely overstimulated by altered food and chemicals that, in many cases, it is our own **antibodies** that are initiating the physical attack against our organs and tissues.[8]

> Note: I have provided additional detail in Part IV on the importance of food and environment as triggers of autoimmunity.

---

[8]   American Autoimmune Related Diseases Association (AARDA)

PART III

Functional Medicine

A NEW MODEL FOR TREATING DISEASE

PROTOCOLS FOR ADRESSING
FUNCTIONAL IMBALANCES

FUNCTIONAL MEDICINE

A New Approach to Todays Health

- Investigates the underlying cause of illness

- Based on Biochemical & Neurological Individuality

- Solutions include Diet, Lifestyle, Advanced Rehab

- Concerned with Long Term Impacts

- Embraces Epigenetics where health is viewed as a combination of Genes and environment

Functional Medicine is looking for a deeper pattern of illness.

The Birth of Functional Medicine

The early work advanced by the Functional Medicine Institute provided much needed frameworks to the victims for the newly emerged "medical business" model. It brought an invitation to "take a moment and get the details right" and see who you were treating and investigate their issues with an expanded diagnostic and therapeutic consciousness.

Organ-based functional medicine started the wellness revolution and is in many ways responsible for the tone, attitude and structure of the modern Functional Movement.

This is not "New Age Medicine". It has **evidence-based researched processes** at its core. It rejects conventional-standard of practice modes of practice in favor of updated research-oriented techniques.

Because of the principal of "**Integrative Medicine" which states that all systems are inter-related**, Functional Medicine looks at the patient analytically according to major systems and further adds "integrative" thinking about their interrelatedness and their impact on the whole person.

Triggers, modulators and preconditions

The first Functional Medicine systems simplistically characterized the diagnostic paradigm as **Antecedents, Triggers and Modulators**.

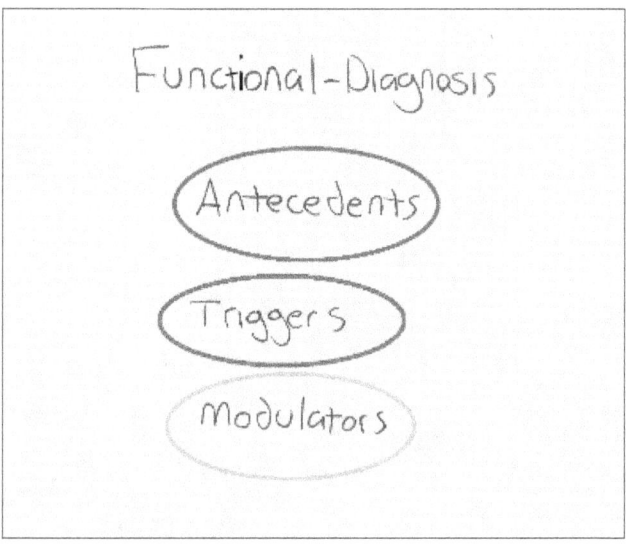

This model has grown in sophistication, acceptance and usefulness to become the newer more complex Functional Medicine trees of interrelationships.

Key systems for investigation of each patient include:

- Structure
- Digestion
- Vasculature
- Daily Life

- Detoxification
- Neurology
- Hormones
- Stress

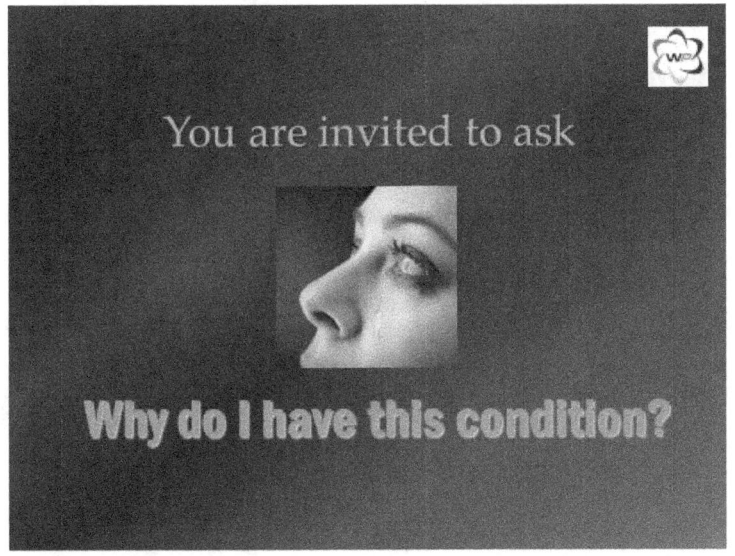

Early functional medicine frameworks forced practitioners to get the whole story behind the diagnosis and significantly improved work on multi-system conditions.

Epigenetics

A key concept coming out of the functional medicine movement is that DNA coding supplies only part of the answer. Genetic expression is seen as a kind of a song being played by an instrument (the DNA code) and the artist (the experiences of life).[9]

> *This "wash of life" across our DNA code is then responsible for our outcomes. There is no assumption of genetic predetermination and medical positivism is reborn. TAS*

The solution to the food and environmental triggers of modern disease is now up to the individual. It is not a new drug. It is not a surgery. Conventional approaches are not going to help you with it.

---

[9] At the writing of the book, we are getting the first wave of true DNA analysis for the public. While these genetic predispositions can be invaluable in understanding how you are constructed, they still only carry half the answer. The decisions we make concerning our food and environment are crucial inputs to the health equation.

This forced some medical practitioners to realize that part of the resolution of environmentally triggered illness is the elimination of poisonous and antigenic foods from our diet and the avoidance of dangerous chemicals, metals, poisons and infection.

Starting with Inflammation, our model adds autoimmunity, chemical and metal toxicity, hormone imbalance, stress and trauma. TAS

Inflammation - Immunity Grids

There was some very good work in the early stages of Functional Medicine that attempted to describe the *balance of health* called homeostasis or homeodynamics.

The idea here is that while these important body processes are necessary for life, too much or too little results in disease processes.

The goal is to dwell in the middle range where your inflammation is reacting to trauma without causing damage of its own and the immune system is keeping things microbe free without attacking your own tissues.

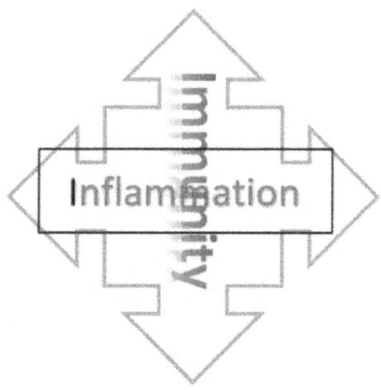

Inflammation is a key vascular function in the healing process. It can be initiated by any stimulus resulting in cell damage. This includes physical and chemical irritants, pathogens and trauma. When we injure any tissue we set an inflammatory cascade in motion.

While crucial to healing, **inflammation** can contribute to the onset of **disease.**

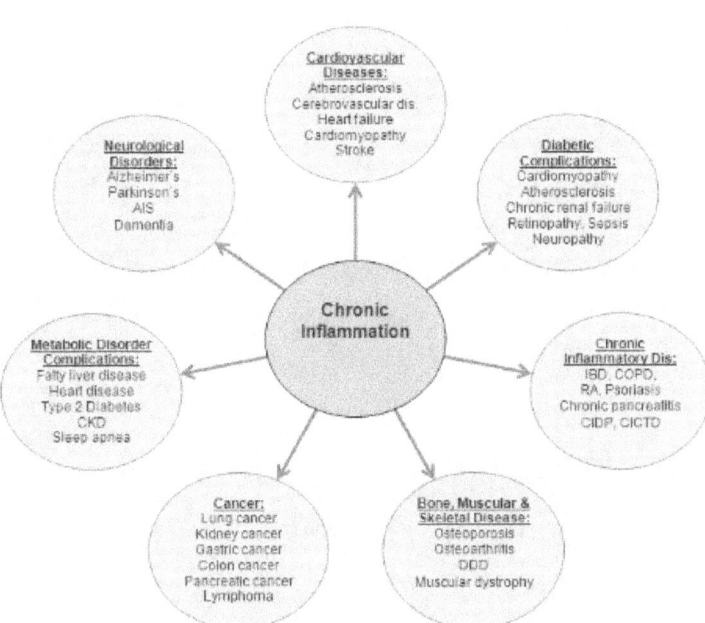

These includes the many inflammatory diseases of our time.:

- Arthritis
- Ankylosing Spondylitis
- Appendicitis
- bronchitis
- Bursitis
- Colitis
- Cystitis

- Dermatitis
- Periodontitis
- Phlebitis
- RSD/CRPS
- Rhinitis
- Tendonitis
- Tonsillitis
- Vasculitis

We can add Coronary Artery Disease, Alzheimer's' Disease and most Cancers to the diseases which likely find their roots in inflammation.

Inflammation is such a key marker for today's diseases that many practitioners think that it is "The Primary Condition" that causes disease.

THE FOUR VECTORS OF HEALTHCARE

Electromagnetic Support
- ✓ Acupuncture
    Laser and Needle
- ✓ Homeopathic Medicine
- ✓ Traditional Chinese Medicine
- ✓ Ayurvedic Medicine
- ✓ Bio-balancing
- ✓ Air and Water Ion Balance
- ✓ Electro-therapies
- ✓ Magnetic Field Therapies
- ✓ Color and Light Therapies

Mental/Emotional Support
- ✓ Guided Imagery
- ✓ Meditation
- ✓ Cognitive Skill Development
- ✓ Homeopathic Medicine
- ✓ Botanical Support
- ✓ Breathing Techniques
- ✓ Stress Reduction Techniques
- ✓ Rescripting Traumas
- ✓ Emotional Release Techniques
- ✓ Aromatherapy, Music, and Sound

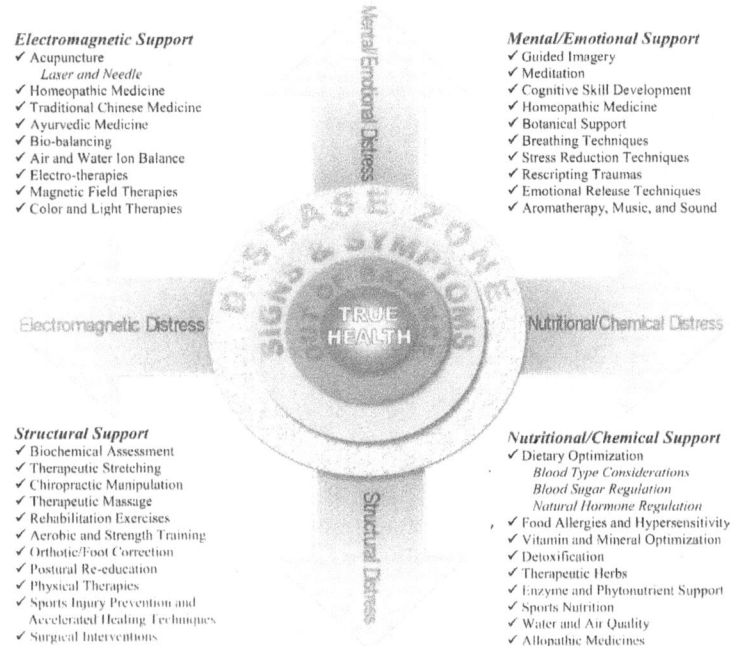

Structural Support
- ✓ Biochemical Assessment
- ✓ Therapeutic Stretching
- ✓ Chiropractic Manipulation
- ✓ Therapeutic Massage
- ✓ Rehabilitation Exercises
- ✓ Aerobic and Strength Training
- ✓ Orthotic/Foot Correction
- ✓ Postural Re-education
- ✓ Physical Therapies
- ✓ Sports Injury Prevention and
    Accelerated Healing Techniques
- ✓ Surgical Interventions

Nutritional/Chemical Support
- ✓ Dietary Optimization
    Blood Type Considerations
    Blood Sugar Regulation
    Natural Hormone Regulation
- ✓ Food Allergies and Hypersensitivity
- ✓ Vitamin and Mineral Optimization
- ✓ Detoxification
- ✓ Therapeutic Herbs
- ✓ Enzyme and Phytonutrient Support
- ✓ Sports Nutrition
- ✓ Water and Air Quality
- ✓ Allopathic Medicines

This early, but comprehensive model balanced
Structure, Chemistry, Emotions and
Electromagnetics *years before their time.*

Immunity

The second process which must be balanced is the body's immune response. We need to monitor both the level and type of reaction.

Too Much Immune Reaction

Increased Immune Response resulting in antibody autoimmune diseases like Thyroid Disease, Ashma, Diabetes, Arthritis, Celiac and Gluten Intolerence, Leukemia and Alzheimer's Disease.

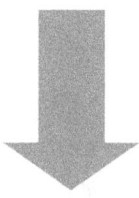

Too Little Immune Reaction

Lowered Immune response resulting in chronic infections and inability to heal.

TH1- TH2 Immune Response

Immunity is also divided according to the type of response the body generates to a given assault.

TH1- The cell-mediated response uses white blood cells to kill pathogens. Th-2 -Antibodies are used in the humeral system and are often the culprits in unexplained autoimmune diseases.

CELL-MEDIATED IMMUNE RESPONSE

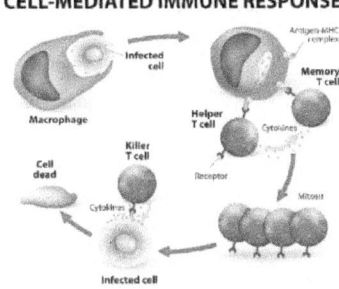

HUMORAL IMMUNITY

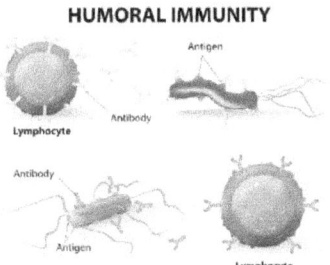

While many times, eliminating the food that triggers the problem, or balancing adrenal, sex or thyroid hormones, or chelating metals and detoxing organs can be effective in quelling immune imbalances. The TH1/TH2 differentiation remains an invaluable tool for balancing immune function.

See the Model for Triggers of Autoimmune Diseases Chart in the next section.

Models to Treat Chronic Disease

(Doing extra to achieve better results)

Today's conventional medicine is about minimizing symptoms. It is surprising to see how little work is being done to actually reverse the disease processes.

There are reliable methodologies which significantly reduce or eliminate symptoms —even in very ill people. These robust frameworks and methods of thinking have provided the basis of Functional Medicine critical thinking.[10]

In most cases, these protocols track the physiology and address each step in the process.

This is an outline for the process we use for complex conditions.

---

[10] Jeffrey Bland, Ph.D. Chief Science Officer, Metagenics President, Metaproteomics Chronic Illness: What Works? Part One: The Four 'R' Program

Step by step Model to reverse Chronic Disease

Chronic Disease is generally considered conventionally untreatable. This is an outline for more effective resolution of chronic disease progression.

Sometimes a simple list is a useful thing. This is much more complex for individual cases, but it give the practitioner key touch points to explore.

1. Understand and **Address the Cause of the Disease** or condition.

2. Balance the level and type of **Immune response**.

3. Balance the Healing or **Inflammatory response** – not too much or too little.

4. **Restore the Cellular reserves**, including antioxidants and chemical components.

5. **Rehabilitate the cells, organs, and body systems** to pre-injury or pre-disease levels.

For Thyroid Conditions, for example, practitioners almost exclusively use a single Hormone marker, **TSH**, to diagnose and track the patient condition.

There is actually a 7-part hormonal cascade originating in the Brain and affecting every cell. We have an epidemic of undiagnosed Thyroid patients in the United States because of this practice.

What is the alternative? We can order more extensive labs that track Hypothalamus function with TRH, Pituitary with TSH, Thyroid gland with T4, the Liver and Small Intestines with their independent varieties of T3, Thyroid Binding Globulin for transportation, and Thyroid Antibodies for autoimmune activity.

Other systems such as Adrenals, Sex hormones and Neurotransmitters are also prospective targets to fully understand the implication of this condition.

Reaching beyond biochemistry, a truly integrative approach could add **functional neuro tests** to see how the brain is performing, and qEEG brains scans to understand Hyper or Hypo neural function for the same condition. The kind of testing performed can have a major impact on the direction of care.

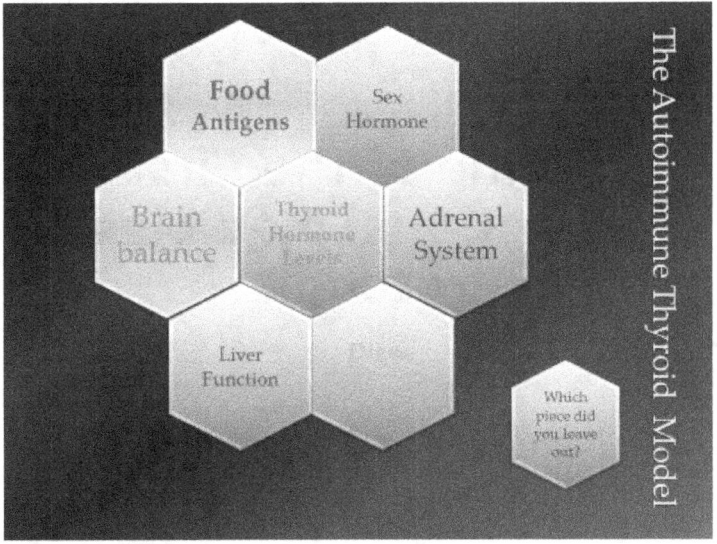

In many cases the testing protocols determine the depth and direction of clinical impression and care. Diversity and level of practitioner training distinguish what level of support the patient receives.

Some of the First Functional Medicine Protocols –

The 4-R protocol for GI Restoration

Remove Replace Reinoculate & Repair

Because the Gut is pivotal in ensuring proper absorption and metabolism, enzyme formation and essential amino acid introduction, it is a primary system for Functional Medicine practitioners.

4-R model was developed to address the details of processes that could go wrong with this important system.

This was one of the first Functinal Medicine formal departures from convention. On the opposite page, I have provided our 15 year old version of our implementation of the 4 R protocol.

While outdated compared to DNA testing and Advanced Amino Acid Analysis, it still outperforms the offhand dietary advice given by most practitioners.

THE WELLNESS PROS — Dr. Thomas A. Santucci, DC, Certified Nutritional Specialist

CDSA Recommendations for _____ Date _____

Four R" Approach to Gastrointestinal Restoration – Remove, replace, reinoculate & repair

Remove: Eradicate any pathogenic microflora, yeast and/or parasites with natural or prescription agents suggested on the CDSA (i.e., berberine/goldenseal, garlic, artemesia, citris seed extract, uva ursi, etc.). Eliminate known allergenic foods and/or follow a modified elimination diet by avoiding dairy and gluten containing foods, and emphasizing fresh nonprocessed foods.

Anti-Bacterial	**Para Biotic Plus** or	___/_____	Duration: _____ weeks
(Anti-bacterial/yeast/virus)	**GI Synergy**	___/_____	Duration: _____ weeks
AntiCandida	**Candibactin AR**	___/_____	Duration: _____ weeks
	Garlic 7000	___/_____	Duration: _____ weeks
↑Immune Func.	**Andrographics**	___/_____	Duration: _____ weeks

Replace: Provide pancreatic multidigestive enzymes and HCL if appropriate, particularly if markers of malabsorption are present on the CDSA.

Digestive Enzymes	**Duozyme**	___/_____	Duration: _____
(HCL)	**Gluten Flam**	___/_____	
	Ultra Gest	___/_____	

Reinoculate: Administer lactobacillus acidophilus, bifidobacteria and probiotics such as fructooligosaccharides (FOS) and inulin.

Pro-Biotic	**Strengtia**	___/_____	Duration: _____
(Good bacteria)	**Pro Flora**	___/_____	
	Ultra Flora	___/_____	

Repair: Provide nutrients to support gastrointestinal mucosal integrity, such as L-glutamine, antioxidants, glutathione, N-acetylcystein (NAC), zinc, pantothenic acid, medium chain triglycerides (MCTs), fiber, etc.

Rebuilding Sm	**Intestinal Repair Caps**	___/_____	Duration: _____ weeks
Intestine	**Intestinal Repair Cmplx**	___/_____	Duration: _____ weeks
	RepairVite	___/_____	Duration: _____ weeks

Liver Rebuild: After intestinal issues have been effectively corrected, upregulation of liver detoxification pathways can be accomplished by providing nutrients which are used in phase I biotransformation and phase II conjugation pathways. These may include individual nutrients such as N-acetyl cysteine, methionine, cysteine, glycine, glutamic acid, glutathione and antioxidant nutrients. However, the use of a specifically designed formulary medicinal food products are much more practical and efficient to use clinically.

Liver	**Methyl SP**	___/_____	Duration: _____ weeks
Detoxification	**Hepatoplex**	___/_____	Duration: _____ weeks
Balance Phase I & II	**Metacrin Dx**	___/_____	Duration: _____ weeks
Detox Pathways			

Copyright The Wellness Pros 07/24/2008
C:\SharedDocs\Office Forms\Current Office Forms\Biochemistry & Nutrition Information\Nutritional Recommendation Forms\CDSA 201C\CDSA Recommendations Sheet.docx

Traditional 4 R Support Protocol

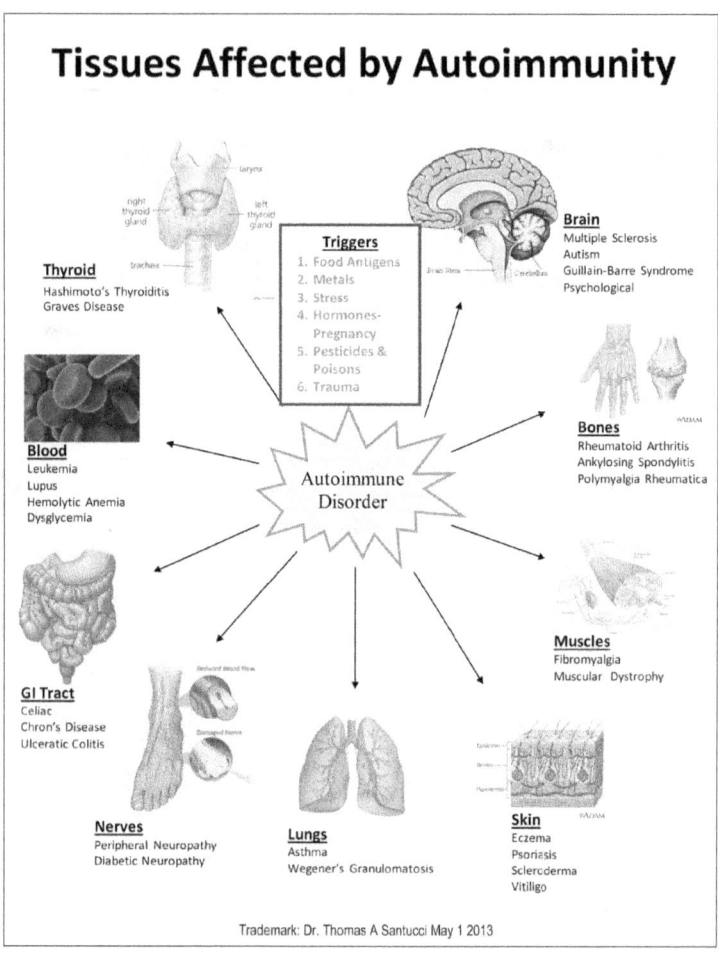

Tissues Affected by Autoimmunity

Triggers
1. Food Antigens
2. Metals
3. Stress
4. Hormones-
   Pregnancy
5. Pesticides &
   Poisons
6. Trauma

Autoimmune Disorder

Thyroid
Hashimoto's Thyroiditis
Graves Disease

Blood
Leukemia
Lupus
Hemolytic Anemia
Dysglycemia

GI Tract
Celiac
Chron's Disease
Ulceratic Colitis

Nerves
Peripheral Neuropathy
Diabetic Neuropathy

Lungs
Asthma
Wegener's Granulomatosis

Skin
Eczema
Psoriasis
Sclercderma
Vitiligo

Brain
Multiple Sclerosis
Autism
Guillain-Barre Syndrome
Psychological

Bones
Rheumatoid Arthritis
Ankylosing Spondylitis
Polymyalgia Rheumatica

Muscles
Fibromyalgia
Muscular Dystrophy

Trademark: Dr. Thomas A Santucci May 1 2013

I developed this chart to illustrate that Autoimmune Diseases are rarely a single set of symptoms. Most Immune patients have multiple named Immune conditions.

PART IV

Autoimmunity

A NEW MODEL FOR
TREATING DISEASE

PROTOCOLS FOR ADRESSING
FUNCTIONAL IMBALANCES

Antibodies and Autoimmune Disease

While today's chronic conditions have many involved organ systems with lots of individual nuances, they usually fall into two broad categories- Environmental or Autoimmune.

Our polluted water, air and food has set us a level of toxicity that overwhelm anything we are programmed to handle. This has supplied the triggers for immune generated self-attacks pervading the "diseases of modern man diagnostics".

In 2010, I made a chart to explain to patients that Thyroid disease, Celiac disease, Rheumatoid arthritis, Peripheral Neuropathy, Anemia, and many brain issues were found together and were very likely the end result of autoimmune activity spurred by predictable antigen sources.

It turns out, that all of these tissues share similar protein immune receptors with the current manipulated wheat molecules.

Food Supply and the Gluten-Intolerance epidemic

Further explaining these diseases, the autoimmune cascade can impact any tissue and can be initiated by any one or multiple triggers. For example, Gluten Intolerance or Arsenic toxicity can both compel the immune system to attack the Thyroid and the Central Nervous System while simultaneously contributing to Anemia and rheumatoid arthritis.

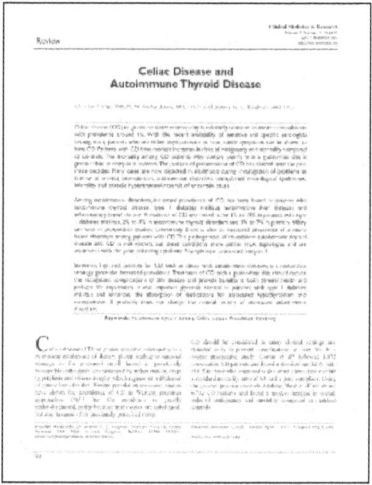

Food

Our Daily Bread is at least partially responsible for the myriad of autoimmune diseases, as well as the avalanche of childhood development problems that is inundating our society.

Why does food cause a problem?

In addition to a primary processor of food, out digestive tracts act as discriminators of the environment and the food we eat. That is, it makes a decision as to whether it is food meant to be eaten and absorbed or is actually a pathogen (bacteria, virus or parasite) and is meant to be killed.

In some cases, the system gets it wrong and attacks food. It turns out the system attacks a **few select foods**, namely **Gluten, dairy, egg, yeast and soy a lot more frequently than most other foods.** The connection is that all of these foods that have been significantly tampered with by their producers.

Testing our Food Sensitivities

It is an unhappy thought that the bread and butter staples we endear are actually harmful and in some cases deadly. Because of this, it has been necessary to develop testing with extremely high reliability to show DNA incompatibility and harmful antibody proliferation. (See list of tests which may benefit you.)

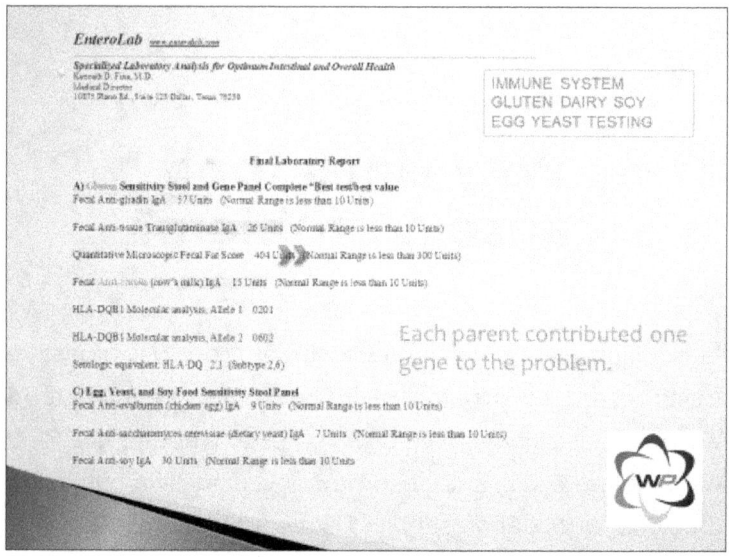

Americans, more than other nationalities, tend to be skeptical when their institutions or prior beliefs are questioned. The story of food manipulation and genetic modification has also been well documented and again, I will not replay it here. Among others, **Grain Brain**, Dr Permutter's, excellent book has done that.

Unfortunately, we have grown to understand antibody provoking foods as a part of the landscape in which we exist. It is like living in a beautiful countryside with land mines.

Clinically, when we are tasked with getting to the bottom of complex conditions, **food is often a starting point (trigger) for the patient's downturn.**

The food news seems incontrovertible. **Wheat, dairy, eggs and soy are seriously suspect in the increase in autoimmune tissue damage.**

ADD/ASD

There is a special kind of epidemic that is affecting us all. An epidemic in the normal development of our children. The subject of attention deficit kids with its seven types of expressive disorders and the range of "kids on the spectrum" has taken us all by storm.

There is a correlation or coincidence in the statistics of Autism and Gluten intolerance. The number of new ASD kids has grown steadily with the new Gluten intolerance cases - both conditions have increased far beyond anything that genetics alone allows.[11]

While there have been many attempts to downplay the numbers, the statistics support the statement that 30% of all 18-year-old males in the United States will develop ADD.

Of equal importance is that this epidemic is at least partly environmental. As of the writing of this book, 100% of the

---

[11] Why is Wheat Gluten Disorder on the Rise? Joseph Mercola, July 23, 2009

ADHD kids in our clinical community have tested with an intolerance to Gluten.

In many cases, the families were not aware of the connection. So the trip to the grocery store is now focused on selecting foods without autoimmune consequences.

"You can't fix what you can't find."

- very old diagnostic adage.

I have included a couple of "What you can do" guides in the next section. These highlight some of the testing used in Functional Medicine.

Note: that there are other good tests like Organic Acid Testing, Metalation tests or Expanded Predictive Antibody testing that can provide even more information. These are the basics.

Getting better answers with Testing

Because we are all biochemically unique we benefit from unique testing. This is a basic list of testing options you can consider.

Blood Chemistry Analysis- Provides foundational work for establishing reserves necessary for good health.

When evaluated against Functional ranges rather than traditional lab values, a robust Blood Chemistry panel can give key insights into **organ function.**

The new **Predictive Antibody DNA panels** take the uncertainty out of allergy testing and shed light on autoimmune food intolerances. Gluten, Dairy, Egg & Soy intolerance have risen 70%. (Test shown in Food section)

Adrenal stress - the modern world is slowly depleting our reserves and spiking Cortisol to disease levels. The adrenal system is one of three key systems that affect all tissues and regularly fail in the course of living our complex lives.

Digestive Testing – The Gut Biome is being reintroduced into the popular consciousness. Testing the 100 Trillion resident bacteria may yield important information on your metabolic and immune functions.

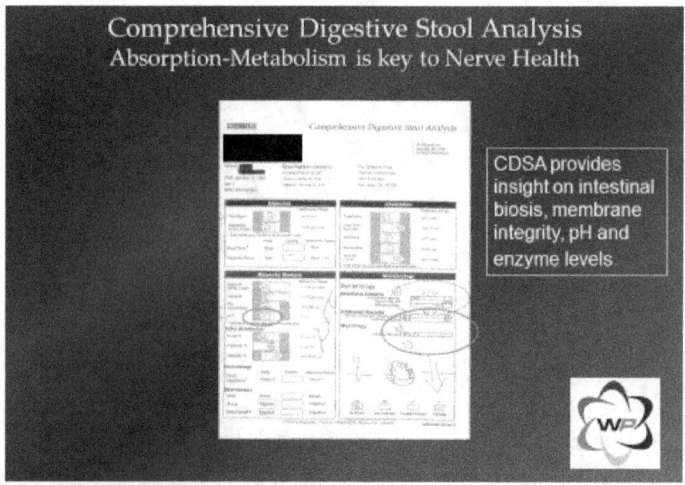

Comprehensive Digestive Stool Analysis
Absorption-Metabolism is key to Nerve Health

CDSA provides insight on intestinal biosis, membrane integrity, pH and enzyme levels.

Metals- Heavy metal testing is used with neuropathy and dementia patients, but is useful for families with well water, anyone who eats food from inland water sources and for international travelers

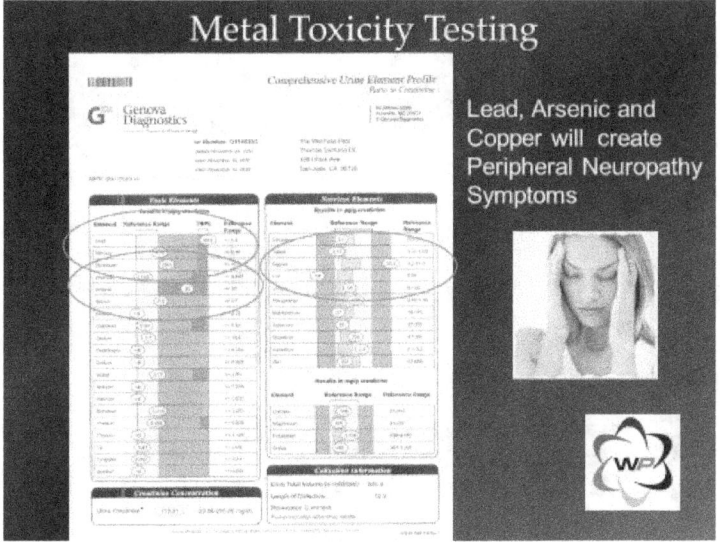

Stimulated Cytokine Testing

This is a little more advanced test which classifies food, supplements and clinical protocols into separate Immune sensitive categories. Green tea is good for some people and bad for others.

Neurotransmitters- your brain runs on 10 key chemicals. How are they doing? It's is an opportunity to safely influence mental performance.

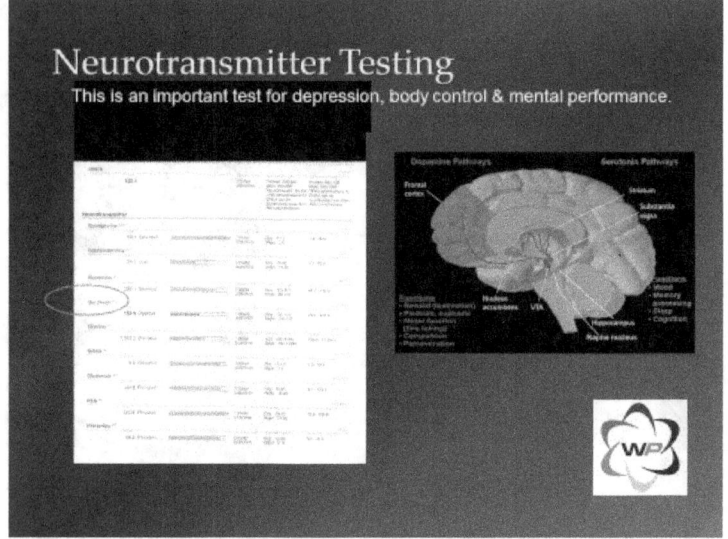

*Advanced testing led us to develop
better natural interventions.
The following 2 charts are representative
protocols we used in the past for nutritional
interventions for many common conditions.*

Natural Intervention

Examples of Supplement Protocols used for clinical support

THE WELLNESS PR?S   Dr. Thomas A. Santucci, DC, Certified Nutritional Specialist

Nutritional Support Recommendations for ....   **Date** ....

Nutritional Goals:

- Food Antigen avoidance - Gluten, Dairy, Soy
- Gut & Brain Barrier Membrane Integrity
- Intestinal Permeability- Support Liver and GALT
- Gut Restoration- Dysbiosis/Yeast/ Enzymes
- Detox metals and pesticides
- Pre/Post Cancer Support
  - Neurotransmitters
  - Adrenal Hormones-Cortisol
  - Female Hormones /Male Hormones
  - Inflammation & Pain
  - Long Term Neuro Protection
    - Cardiac Protection

Modifications: **Gluten** Dairy Eggs Yeast Soy   Decrease: Plastic Contact   Preservatives   Electronics
Add: Pink Salt   Olive Oil   Coconut Oil   Vegetable Juicing   Aloe Pro   Dense Protein

Daily Nutritional Support:

Multi Vitamin	Maxum II IV /. B-Max	____/x per meal	Duration:	Ongoing
Digestive Enzymes	Premier HCl / HCl Activator	____/x per meal	Duration:	Ongoing
	Digestase/Gluten Flam/CM Core	____/x per meal	Duration:	Ongoing
EPA/DHA	Ortho Omega/ BioOmega 369 Emulsion	____/2x daily	Duration:	Ongoing(Cell Membr)
Vitamin D3	Premier D3 Drops	____/2x daily	Duration:	Ongoing (Immune)
Vitamin E	Premier Deltanol Tocotrienol	____/2x daily	Duration:	Ongoing (Fat Liver)
Antioxidants	Vit C / IP6/Tumeric /CoQ10/Ubiq / Glutathione Rec/ Oxicell	____/2x daily	Duration:	Ongoing(your choice)
Probiotics	PRL/ Strengthia/ Pro Flora	____/2x daily	Duration:	Ongoing
Anti-inflammatory	EFAC/ Bio Inflammatory	____/x daily	Duration:	
Pain	Pain-X / Inflamazyme / Bromlaj	____/2x daily	Duration:	Ongoing

Optional Add-on Vit A, VICO, EFAC, Oxicell, Hbi6, Enzimes, DHA, Glutathione Recicler, anti-inflammatories, Anemia, Blood Sugar, Thyroid, Int'l, Muscle, Adl, Biere 3

Blood Support:

Insulin Resistance	PRL/Glysen/Protoglysen	____/____	Duration:	____weeks
Hypoglycemia	**Proglyco-SP**	____/____	Duration:	____weeks
Blood Iron	**HemeVite/ PRL**	____/____	Duration:	____weeks
B Vit Anemia	**Max-B, B6, B12, B1, B2, B3**	____/____	Duration:	____weeks
Energy/Circulation	Nitric Balance	____/____	Duration:	____weeks

Adrenal Support:

Adrenals	Adrenal Support +/ **AdreCor**	____/____	Duration:	____weeks
HPA Axis	**Adaptocrine / AdrenaCalm**	____/____	Duration:	____weeks
Adrenal Support	**Adrenastim**	____/____	Duration:	____weeks

Digestion Repair:

GI Repair	**GI Revive / DFH Program**	____/____	Duration:	____days
	RepairVite ClearVite	____/____	Duration:	____days
Probiotics	**PRL/ Strengthia/ Pro Flora**	____/____	Duration:	____weeks
Anti-bacterials	PRL/ GI Synergy /ParaBiotic Plus	____/____	Duration:	____weeks
Anti-Viral	Green Olive Leaf/ Immune upregulator	____/____	Duration:	____weeks
Anti-Parasitic	**Paratosin**			
Anti-yeast	**PRL/Garlic7000/Candibactin**	____/____	Duration:	____weeks
Constipation	Dr Shulz #1/LuxaGen / Aloe Pro / Physllium Husk			

Sleep/Circadian Rhythm Support:

Sleep Cycle	Kavanace PM/Sleep Factors	____/____	Duration:	____weeks
Melatonin	**Tranquinol/ Serotone**	____/____	Duration:	____weeks
	Vitamin B12 / Methyl-SP	____/____	Duration:	____weeks

Nutrition Interventions Options

Detoxification (Also see separate Instruction Sheets)

Liver/GB Cleanse	Tomato/Olive Oil/Turmeric/ Allicidin	_____ / x weekly	Duration: _____	months
Coffee Flush	Coffee/Aloe/ _____	_____ / x weekly	Duration: _____	months
Master Flush	Lemon Juice/ etc	_____ / x weekly	Duration: _____	months
Castor Oil Packs.	Premier castor Oil/ wool fleece/ Hot Pack Cation packs/ dental Packs.			

Liver Detoxification Support:

Liver	Liver NP / HepataVen/	___/_____	Duration: _____ weeks
Detoxification GB	**BileVen/ Bilemin**	___/_____	Duration: _____ weeks
Balance Phase I & II	**Metacrin Dx**	___/_____	Duration: _____ weeks

Autoimmune Support:

Autoimmune Goals.
1) Manage severity of autoimmune flare ups. 2) Minimize autoimmune activity by balancing antigenic response (manage the food triggers).
3) Identify all affected tissues of the autoimmune reaction- thyroid, brain, GI tract, blood, skin, bones, lungs. etc.

Immune Balance	Ultra D Complex/ D3		Duration: _____ weeks
TH1 Support	**X-Viromin/Ecinacia/ (List)**	___/_____	Duration: _____ weeks
TH2 Support	Reservatrol/**X-FLM/ Coffee / (List)**	___/_____	Duration: _____ weeks
Immune Support	Allimax - Andrographics		Duration: _____ weeks
	Nitric Ox		Duration: _____ weeks

Neurotransmitter Support:

General Brain	Acetyl-CH	___/_____	Duration: _____ weeks
	Methyl-SP/ B12	___/_____	Duration: _____ weeks
Daily Support	**Stress X**	___/_____	Duration: _____ weeks
Memory	Cognifactors/ Membrane	___/_____	Duration: _____ weeks
Serotonin	**Serotone**	___/_____	Duration: _____ weeks
Dopamine	**Dopatone**	___/_____	Duration: _____ weeks
GABA	**Gabatone**	___/_____	Duration: _____ weeks
NeuroAdrenal	**Balance D**	___/_____	Duration: _____ weeks
Brain balance.	**Avipaxin.**	___/_____	Duration: _____ weeks
_____	_____	___/_____	Duration: _____ weeks

Brain-Immune Support:

Neuro Inflammation	NeuroFlam (Brain Fog)	___/_____	Duration: _____ weeks
Blood Flow	NeurO2	___/_____	Duration: _____ weeks
	Nitric Oxide	___/_____	Duration: _____ weeks
Antioxidant	Glutathione Rec.	___/_____	Duration: _____ weeks

Brain Barrier Support:

Fatty Acids	**Phyto Brain-E**	___/_____	Duration: _____ weeks
	Brain-E	___/_____	Duration: _____ weeks

Female Support:

Headaches	**MigraPlex/ Migramax**	___/_____	Duration: _____ weeks
Hot Flashes	**EstroFactors**	___/_____	Duration: _____ weeks
H. Imbalances	**Phytobalance**	___/_____	Duration: _____ weeks

Thyroid Gland Support: Brain/Pituitary Support:

Natural Support	Thyroxal	___/_____	Duration: _____
	Thyro-Zyme	___/_____	Duration: _____
Pituitary Support	**Thyraxis PT**	___/_____	Duration: _____ weeks
Adrenal Support	**Adaptocrine**	___/_____	Duration: _____ weeks
	Adrenacalm	___/_____	Duration: _____ weeks
Under Conversion	**Thyro CNV**	___/_____	Duration: _____ weeks
	Oxicell	___/_____	Duration: _____ weeks
Rx Support by MD	**HRT**	to be prescribed by your Primary Care Physician	

Page 2 - Nutrition Support Protocols

Six dietary changes that can really make a difference (To Do List)

We all have two part-time jobs.
The first is to not get Heart Disease and the
Second is to not get Cancer.

By eliminating food antigens,
balancing blood sugar, alkalizing our
chemistry and supplying our nervous systems
with essential nutrients, we can go a long way
toward meeting these responsibilities.

Dr Santucci

Manage your blood sugar. Consistent levels of blood glucose are responsible for proper energy & mood, cardiac health and optimal neurologic status. Spikes in insulin are unfailingly destructive to neural tissue.

Acidifying your stomach — a low gastric pH provides the chemical power to cleave protein molecules, protects you from food borne infection and most likely prevent infection originated cancer.

Alkalize the rest of you — Because the stomach absorbs proteins and alcohols (and not carbs) juicing provides the best conduit to introduce alkaline foods to the system.

Balance your Neurotransmitters - Eat enough *essential amino acids* to feed your neurotransmitter requirement. This is best accomplished with a high quality protein food. If you have elected not to eat animal protein you must take definitive steps to augment amino acids.

Avoid GMO foods - We have changed the fundamentals of our food's DNA with potentially disastrous consequences. The genetic modifications do not look like they will be safe for our species.

Absolutely do not eat wheat. It really looks like wheat prompts the body to generate antibodies that start immune attacks against multiple organs. Most of the Hashimoto's Thyroiditis, Chronic Fatigue Syndrome, Fibromyalgia and multiple system autoimmune conditions are fueled by gluten.

PART V

Functional Neurology

RESEARCH-BASED NEUROPATHWAY
BREAKTHROUGHS

REDEFINING INCURABLE
NEURO DISEASES

Conventional Neurology

Probably no other branch of health care is there so much **upside potential** *as neurologic interventions for chronic conditions. With a diagnostic paradigm that generally recognizes progressive conditions in their last, often incurable, stages and the use of drugs and surgery as their primarily tools, neurologists have one of the lowest patient and physician satisfaction levels in medicine.*

One can hope that this situation can only get better, as patient awareness of the enormous potential of this field helps direct a new standard of practice.

Neurogenesis

A key concept coming out of the functional neurology is that the **nervous system can repair itself.** Coupled with the concept of Neurogenesis, it meant that now the old idea of **"permanent" neurological damage** could be clinically challenged.[12]

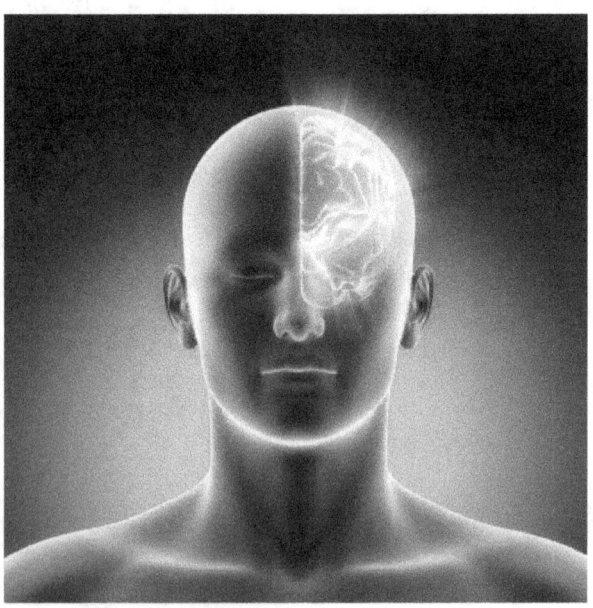

---

[12] David Perlmutter, M.D.
     Neurogenesis: How to Change Your Brain

The New (Functional) Neurology

Functional Neurology revolutionized the diagnosis and support of many brain and nervous system diseases. Weakness, Vertigo, neuropathies, pain, and even the neurodegenerative conditions like Alzheimer's, Parkinson's and dementia have been curtailed and, in some cases, resolved. Patients have regained strength and restored mental function to unprecedented levels.

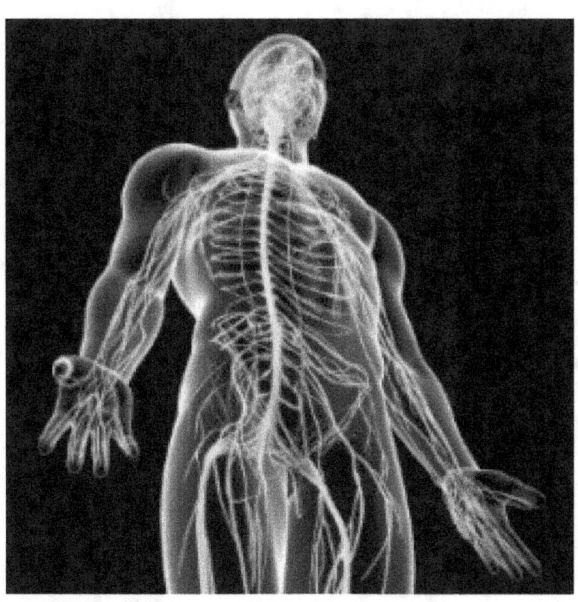

What changed?

20 years ago, Frederic Carrick and a group of researchers initiated a new branch of health care focused on **functional rather than ablative or physical lesions**. Up to that point, Neurologists were primarily concerned with physical lesions which actually destroyed brain or peripheral nerve tissues and could be seen and measured on a CAT scan or MRI.

Functional lesions can be far more subtle and represent neurological problems that are due to dysfunctions of nerve pathways that usually do not show up on scanning technology.

Carrick's Functional Neurology brought the diagnostics of subtle lesions to the 20th century. It required practitioners to "go back to school" and learn a much more involved version of neurophysiology than had previously existed.

Instead of memorizing a handful of neuro pathways for the purpose of passing the MCATs or the Neuro boards, Carrick's doctors attempted to deeply understand 50 to 100 neuro pathways in order to develop a diagnostic paradigm known as the *longitudinal level of the lesion*. This was a kind on neurological triangulation to identify where on the neuro axis the patient's problem was centered.

Comprehensive Neurological & Physical Examination

A thorough and comprehensive exam pinpoints the source of the problem.
LLL –Answers where is the problem on the neuroaxis

Sensory Exam – (Nerve Root Reporting)
Motor Function Exam (Myotomes point to spinal level involved)
Cranial nerve tests – Face & Neck (Mes/Pons/Medulla)
Dorsal Column Testing for WDA Nerve Dysfunction
Tests for balance and coordination (cerebellum) Heart rate/rhythm
Pulse OX (tissue oxygen saturation)
Blood pressure/pulse rate (Brain stem)
Deep Tendon Reflexes (Spinal Cord)

The New Neurological Exam

While technology such as brain scanning functional MRI is now available, Functional Neurology's advanced assessment is primarily being accomplished with a more sophisticated version of the neurological exam.

The new exam brought an improved understanding of how was the brain is actually affecting the sensory and motor systems.

This is accomplished by investigating the patterns of the body's impulses, the contributions of individual lobes, the modifications of sensation and motion by the thalamus and the cerebellum.

Neurologic Screening Examination

R / L **R / L**
Cerebellum Cerebrum

Patient Name _____

Rhomberg's sign *(midline cerebellum)* **Georges Test** – (arterial insuffic)
____ Normal (no sway)   SX____ None ____
____ Abnormal sway Back and Forth or falling RIGHT or LEFT (CB)

Finger to Nose *(parietal with no terminal tremor)* *(cerebellum with terminal tremor)*
Index Finger
____ Normal (touch finger to nose with no difficulty)
____ Abnormal RIGHT or LEFT
Digit 5 Finger
____ Normal (touch finger to nose with no difficulty)
____ Abnormal RIGHT or LEFT

Oxygen Profusion
RT | L
Sp O2 _____
Pulse Pressure _____
Pulse _____ | Quality ____

Past Pointing *(parietal and intermediate cerebellum)*
____ Normal
____ Abnormal RIGHT or LEFT

Rapid Alt Movement: Piano Coordination *(lateral CB)*
____ Normal   ____ Abnormal RIGHT or LEFT

Optokinetic Testing *(Frontal/ Parietal/ Mes /CB)*
Pursuits _____   Saccades _____
_____ Left to Right (Initiation/ Accuracy/ Speed)
_____ Right to Left (Initiation/ Accuracy/ Speed)
_____ Inferior to Superior (Initiation/ Accuracy/ Speed)

Myotome Testing (muscle strength)

	RT	L
C5		
6		
7		
8		
T1		
L1		
L3		
L5		

Collicular Mapping (Superior Colliculus lesion)
Standing with eyes closed
____ Return from RIGHT / LEFT

Joint Position Sense   Digit Span   2 Pt Discrimination
Finger: Rt Left   Fingers: Rt Left Arm: Rt Left Leg: Rt left
Toe: Rt Left
Frontal Lobe Memory recall: "Dog, Paris, Purple" 7 Digit
Recall: Right=Mono Left=Prosodic

Accommodation: Near Vision Testing
____ Normal (eyes converge toward nose)
____ Abnormal right: no convergence /Exophoria
____ left: no convergence /Exophoria
Reflexes (0-5) Lower is LMN Increase is UMN
DTR - Biceps Triceps Brachioradialis
DTR - Patella Achilles Hamstring

Vibration Sensitivity – Periph N.
Shoulder ____ Wrist ____
Upper leg ____ Ankle ____
Trigeminal Nerve Distribution →

V1
V2
V3

Position Sense - 50 Step Test

Corneal Blink -Spontaneous Eyelid Twitch:CN X

Yes R L **No** Eyes should blink & tear bilaterally
Photophobia *(CN III)* ____ Yes ____ No

Doctor Signature: _____

____ Ft Forward – Otoliths
(Remediation is Near-Far Thumbs)

____ Degrees Off –Ipsi Cortex
(Remediation is Non-Linear Complex Motion)

Date _____

News Metabolic Unit   Page 1 of 1   WP Series Screen April 30 2012
Remediation: NLCM on CB Side   Near Far   Neuro Improvement: _____

Functional Neurological Screening Examination

I have an aversion to books filled with patient histories, but in this case I would like to share a file which illustrates the potential in non-drug neurologically based intervention.

The Patient Story

Jean did not cook; she could not drive or leave the house by herself. Jean couldn't carry her own purse because of the pain and fatigue. Jeans husband did all that. Two people's lives were completely consumed with her pain.

Jean had been taking pharmaceutical pain medications for 20 years. Jean woke up every morning and took opioid drugs to lower her constant pain levels to the point that she could bath. She took another set of pain killer to make it to breakfast and another to get dressed.

Jean's Initial Presentation

Jean's neurological examination revealed a significant hemispheric imbalance in the processing performance between her **left and right lobe of her Cerebrum.**

This is the newest and most sophisticate part of the brain and is thought to manage everything from cognition to self-control. It is also a key moderator of the body's normal mitigation of pain signals.

Neurologically, nociceptive or pain messages are constantly generated by the body. Under normal circumstances, they are intercepted and neutralized by the frontal lobe. In this case, Jean's frontal lobe had lost this pain management capability and so she lived in almost constant pain and discomfort.

Therapeutic Outcome

- Jean was given inputs to the Right side of her cortex, consisting of cervical adjustments, Optokinetic stimulation, rehab exercises and blue tinted glasses to moderate the light stimulus to her brain.

- After 5 weeks, her pain levels we're reduced to 50% of her prior levels. In the next ten weeks, she was feeling normal for the first time in 20 years.

Note: This was accomplished without drugs or nerve surgery - but rather by balancing the brain and training the body. This work was done over 15 years ago.

By reestablishing the neurological control typically exercised by the neocortex over the pain signals, she was able to stop the need for opioid medications.

Much of the discussion so far has been a chronicle of the first 50 years of Functional Medicine and Functional Neurology.

Because this section deals with some of the **newest advances in clinical care**, it is oriented more to computers, electronics and energy fields.

But even in the world of high tech, the **tenants of functional medicine are required to obtain a complete picture of the patient condition.**

Note: I have spent some time on the technical details of Neurofeedback and Pulsed Electromagnetic Field Therapies because I believe that these technologies have significant potential to re-create modern Neuropsychological and Physiological rehab.

PART VI

Energy/Technical Medicine

LASERS
NEUROFEEDBACK
FREQUENCY AS MEDICINE

This is a partial list of some important technological and energy-based rehab modalities.

There are many others and each of them could warrant its own book.

There are other extremely hi-tech solutions being developed that are beyond my current level of understanding.

Brain Scans and Neurofeedback

50 years ago the first electro-diagnosticians measured the tiny amounts of electricity allowed through the human skull in an attempt to understand brain function.

This has grown in sophistication to modern EEG systems which amplify and sensitively filter information comparing output data to large fMRI databases.

The outcome of this measurement is a **Brain Map** which allow us to have detailed conversations about level of **Anxiety, Depression, Memory Loss, Sleep issues and ADHD**.

We are able to sort brainwaves generated by the different functional centers of the brain by their respective brain wave speed, typing them as **Delta, Theta, Alpha and Beta waves. So the activity of the Brain is now digitized.**

Brain Scan Explanations- 30 Watts of Power

Magnitude Indicates the Power of the brainwaves generated by Pyramidal cells

Delta	Theta	Alpha	Beta
2-4 Hz - Sleep	4-8 Hz - Limbic	8-12 Hz - Thalamus	12-30 Hz - Frontal
Deep Sleep	Memory	Emotions -"Feel Good" Wave	Cognition
BS & CB	Emotional – Limbic	Affect -Routine activities-	Communication
	Focus	"Brakes of the Brain"	Learning
	Attention	Inner Environment Calmness -Brain at Rest <-Serotonin	Executive Functions
	Brain Stem Functions		

Low

Delta	Theta	Alpha	Beta
Inadequate DHA	Poor Focus	Low motivation	Learning difficulties
(Need Omega 3)	Distractibility	No Energy	Lack of Cognition
	Memory Issues	"Inability to Idle"	Extreme Low – Asperger's
	Emotional Escapes	Impulsive	

High

Delta	Theta	Alpha	Beta
Brain Fog	Difficulty controlling attention and emotions	Anger	Anxiety
Slowing of the Brain		Hyper-emotionality	OCD
Brain Trauma	"Driving with brakes on" not smooth operation	Difficulty controlling emotion	Over-Processing
	Increases Theta is hallmark of ADD		Insomnia
			ADHD

Dominant Frequency

Low Alpha in Dominant Frequency can be indicative of Metabolic Concerns

Connectivity

Demonstrates level of inter - hemisphere communication across the corpus collossum.
High indicates over communicating – a Communication Traffic Jam. Causes slow processing

Asymmetry

Delta in **Right** indicates Emotional concerns. Delta in **Left** indicates cognitive issues	Theta in **Right** indicates insomnia. Theta in **Left** indicates organizational issues	Alpha in Left indicates Depression	Beta in Right indicates Anxiety

The Wellness Pros -2014 NeuroIntegratative Care of Silicon Valley ™

Brain Wave Associated Conditions
and Entrainment Worksheet

Because these results are numeric in quantified EEG, they can then be compared with the results of large populations of individuals with known conditions. **Neurological and psychological diagnosis are now objectified**.[13]

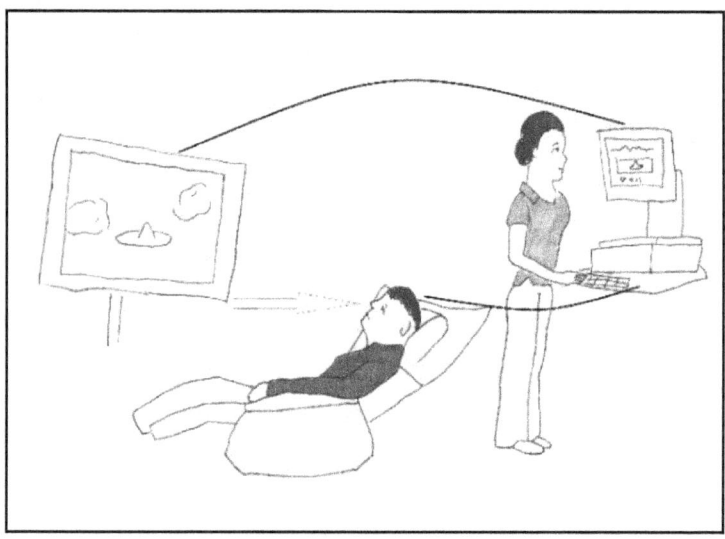

Neurofeedback changes brain frequencies without chemical or direct neurological intervention.

The process of correction is called neurofeedback and brain **entrainment** and involves selecting correcting frequencies to offset over accelerated or slow brain waves.

---

[13] 29. Small JG: Psychiatric disorders and EEG, in Electroencephalography: Basic Principles, Clinical Applications, and Related Fields, edited by Niedermeyer E, Lopes Da Silva F. Baltimore, Williams and Wilkins, 1993, pp 581–596

The significance of this cannot be underestimated. Brain scan now objectify Neurological and psychological conditions. Combined with responsible Neurometabolic interventions, Brain Scans and Neurofeedback offer the promise of greatly improved outcomes for Concussions, Dementia, ADD, Insomnia and Drug Dependence.

Neurofeedback provides fast tangible improvements in Dementias, Trauma, Developmental Delays and emotional imbalances. This is the stuff of the future with the potential to create new nerve pathways in real time.

The New Energy Medicine

Energy Healing - Technology has taken over in this newest and oldest realm of healing.

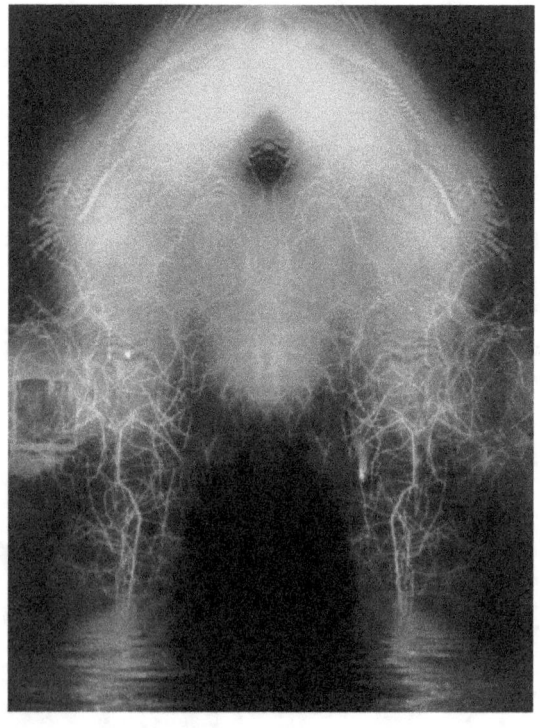

Egyptian Mummy's Energy Field

Frequency modulation, vibration and resonance have been an important part of traditional healing.

New energetic modalities have allowed us to take what was once viewed as a vague *feeling* into numbers on a computer. By understanding and controlling frequency we have the opportunity to turn modulated energy into a source of therapeutic support.

Note:

PEMF is still virtually unknown in modern rehab circles. When we discuss new technologies like this with many of our medical colleagues, we are met with a cautious non-acceptance.

"If anything was this good – why haven't I heard about it?" I have spent time here on the technical description of PEMF to illustrate the level of research and clinical maturity on this important new modality.

Pulsed Electromagnetic Healing

Pulsed Electro Magnetic Force or PEMF is an important new therapy because of its almost universal utility in rehab.

PEMF can reverse micro trauma by repairing the cell membrane and recharging the cell.

Imagine the environment in which your cells exist. A tiny world of cell membranes, organelles, chemical gates and electrical currents. By shunting positively charged sodium and negatively charged potassium ions in and out of the cell, this intelligent cell membrane is responsible for maintaining the integrity of this basic building block of our bodies.

PEMF can be tuned to replicate a powerful version of the earth's **Schumann Waves**. These are electromagnetic waves surrounding the globe which created a steady field with a pulsating 7.83 hertz frequency.

The importance of Schumann waves is evidenced by the fact that students deprived of Schulman waves became sick and despondent when kept in an insulated environment in his early experiments.

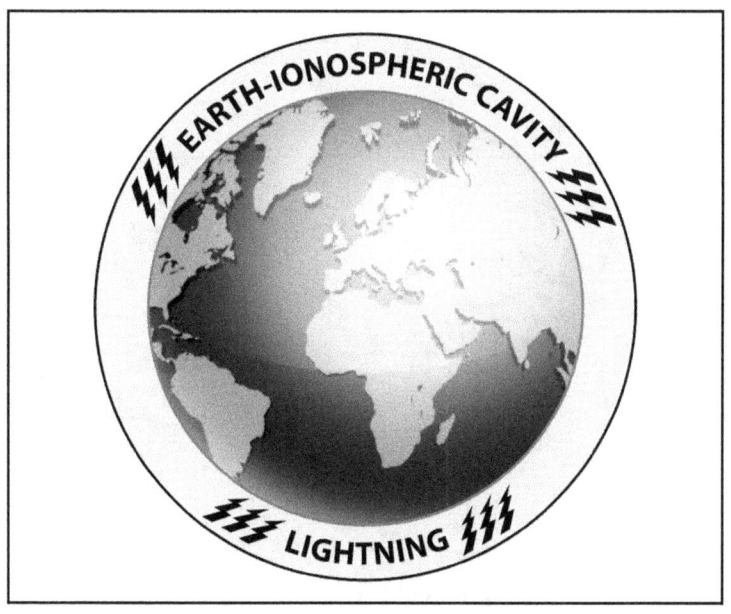

Schumann waves are the result of Lightning
hitting the earth 10-100x a second.

7.83 is the same frequency as the brain's Alpha waves.
Our normal psychological function requires Schuman waves.

We know that the cell membrane integrity is compromised in the cases of ageing, micro-trauma and cancer. So instead of the normative minus 70 mV, the cell is now at minus 50 or minus30 or minus 10 mV. At some critical level, the cell will no longer be responsive to stimulus and will slow down its biological functions.

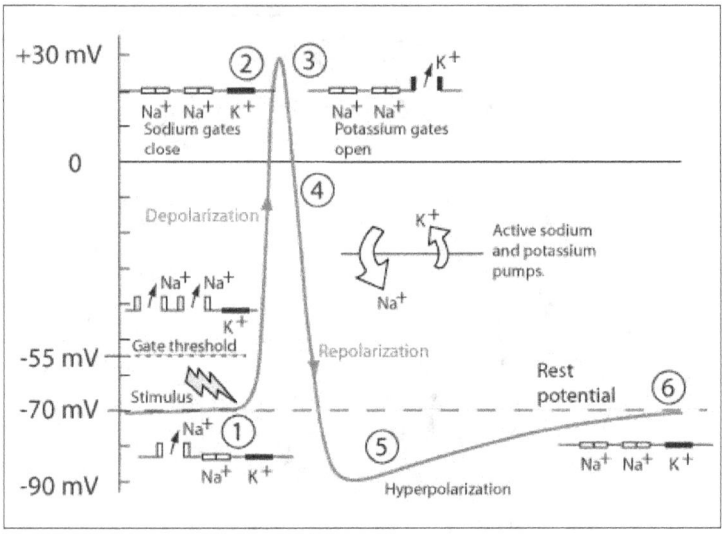

PEMF supplies a high level of naturally occurring ions which energize the cell. These ions also help to maintain the cell membrane in an optimal electric state. By maintaining a -70 mV resting membrane threshold, this cell keeps its shape and healthy viability.

The benefits of PEMF flow from the recharging of the cell and the reestablishment of the cell membrane energy gradient.

Impact on Cellular Environments

Our cells contain electrically charged ions which cause a natural electrical current to flow throughout our body, changes in this current result in activation of key ion pumps which determine the **metabolic rate of the cell**.

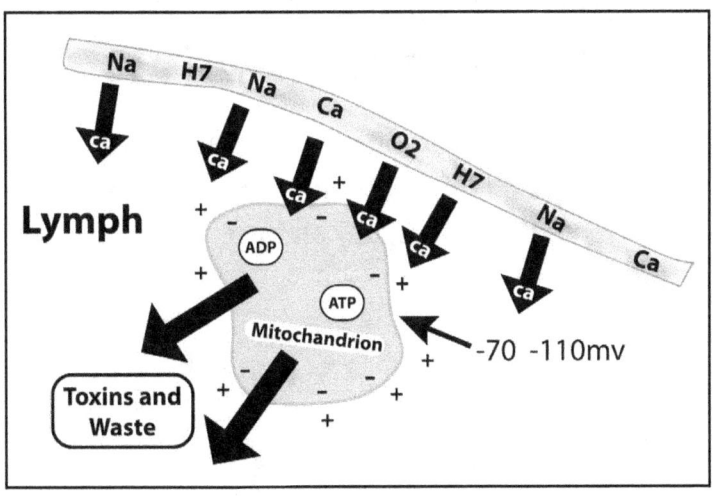

Pulsed Electromagnetic Generators provide energy for the cell to make ATP

What are some of the basic beneficial actions PEMFs will have in my body?

PEMF's ion contribution has a number of physiological effects. It has the capacity to charge red blood cells and increase circulation and oxygenation to cells.

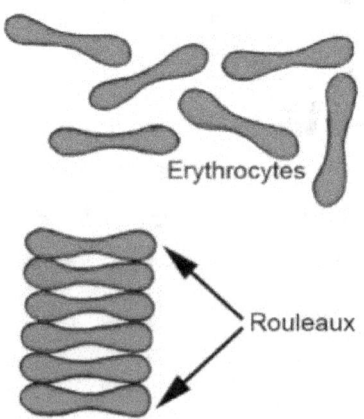

Erythrocytes

Rouleaux

There are multiple experiments where deoxygenated cell in a *Rouleaux formation* have been energized and properly charged allowing the cells to repel themselves and flow normally.

Improved circulation increases the amount of oxygen delivered for healing, regeneration and performance.

Not surprisingly, PEMF has a positive effect on **energy**. The Actin-Myosin mechanism requires fuel for muscle contraction. This takes the form of adenosine triphosphate or ATP.[14] The organ in our cells responsible for converting glucose to ATP is the **mitochondria**. Many Chronic Fatigue patients have mitochondrial performance issues. PEMF works directly on the Mitochondrial DNA and increases cellular output.

Remember in the Functional Medicine section when we discuss the role of inflammation in health and healing? PEMF has an important contribution is reducing inflammation and therefore decreasing healing time.

Research shows us that PEMFs can induce the **proper death** of aged, chronic T lymphocytes, by actions on T cell membranes and key enzymes in cells. For example, PEMFs affect ion flow through specific cell membrane channels (like those for sodium, potassium, and calcium), which positively affects appropriate cell death.

PEMF also has some specific health claims on bone healing. The penetration characteristics allow EMF field to access the living bone and add energy to the repair process.

---

[14] PEMF page 120 - The Fifth Element of Health: Learn Why Pulsed Electromagnetic Field ... By Bryant A. Meyers

PEMF machines are FDA registered for non-union bone fractures, migraine headaches and macular degeneration. Correcting these conditions requires a deep penetration and **significant influence on the cells of the body**.

LASERS - Low Light Emission Lasers

Lasers have been used in physical rehab for 20 years. They should be old hat by now. This is one of the technologies which has not become mainstream despite a preponderance of evidence of their efficacy.

The FDA has registered and cleared low light lasers for muscle pain, back pain, carpel tunnel syndrome and acceleration of wound healing. NASA and US Olympic training coaches have endorsed lasers in their medical and athletic training. LLLT is also the therapy of choice for many difficult pain management challenges such as fibromyalgia and myofascial pain.

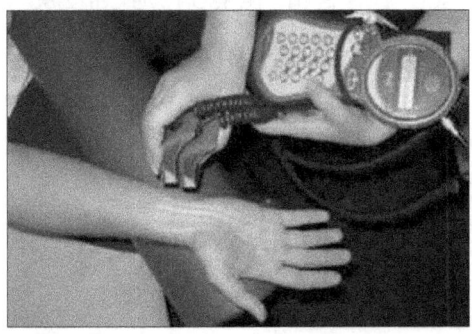

Lasers provide photons that decrease inflammation and increase healing.

Why do lasers work?

Lasers are accelerated light whose photons are dispersed in a **coherent or ordered pattern**. By comparison, light from the sun is not coherent because is diverges in a radiating or random pattern.

Remember that light is both a wave and a particle. The wave form of the laser has the capability to create **resonance or vibration**.

This resonance can be tuned to create specific tones or vibrations which can be used to create changes in living tissues.

Light is also a particle – namely a photon. A photon is much smaller than an electron and has a **far greater penetrating capability** in living tissue. This is the reason we can use it to deliver modulated energy deep within the body.

Lasers decrease inflammation, probably repair DNA and definitely accelerate healing.

Laser effects on human tissue

Lasers reduce Reactive Oxygen Species (ROS) in the same way that metabolic antioxidants work. It is now established that the light at the proper wavelength repairs mitochondrial DNA (mDNA) and messenger RNA (mRNA), used to support and direct maintenance and metabolism in the cell.[15]

> So, at the organ level, these effects combine to heal tissue and promote proper metabolism and function.

---

[15] Lasers Med Sci. 2013 Jul;28(4):1077-84. doi: 10.1007/s10103-012-1191-3. Epub 2012 Sep 2.
DNA repair gene expression in biological tissues exposed to low-intensity infrared laser.
de Souza da Fonseca A1, Mencalha AL, Araújo de Campos VM, Ferreira Machado SC, de Freitas Peregrino AA, Geller M, de Paoli F.

Energy/Technology

In the two years it took to finalize this book, we have seen the introduction of Kaatsu computerized Tourniquet systems for muscle performance, PEMF merged with Neurofeedback equipment and lasers with modulating energy fields added to decompression and neuropathy devices.

We are waiting for improved Brain digitizers, self-tuning energy generators and personal real-time predictors for illness and disease.

Because technology has the potential to bypass some level of the medical intransience by going directly to the consumer, we should all be attentive to the breakthroughs promised by this avenue.

Conclusion

This is a tough subject to compress, even superficially, because the body of knowledge is changing so quickly. Innovations in Biochemistry, Neurology and Energetics keep the solutions coming at top speed.

At the writing of this book, we find ourselves in the presence of new DNA testing, revised detoxification protocols, expansion of predictive antibodies and a dizzying portfolio of equipment changes.

As to the future, it is clear that there is a growing consciousness for patient centered care and equally clear that there are players within health care system intent on maintaining the status quo.

It is my hope that these Neurometabolic Functional Medicine changes are not lost and provide a starting point for the next phase of Effective health interventions which may significantly contribute to human vitality & life span.

What is next

*Finalizing this history has prompted me to start work on the political side of not just affordable, but **Effective,** Health Care Protocols.*

*I am envisioning the **Association for Responsible Medicine** (ARM) to reexamine the scientific basis of care protocols which comprise the iconic*

"Standard of Practice" which get practitioners paid and protected. There is a great deal of struggle and good which may come from this.

*On a less stressful level, I think that the work on the comic, **Functional Medicine in a Fictitious World** needs to come to light so that some of the more penetrating issues of healthcare can be openly discussed.*

Thomas Santucci

Reference List

Atalay, S., Coruh, A., & Deniz, K. (2014). Stromal vascular fraction improves deep partial thickness burn wound healing. *Burns: Journal of the International Society for Burn Injuries*.

Bland, J. (2009, September 10). Chronic Illness: What Works? Part One: The Four 'R' Program. The Huffington Post. Retrieved from http://www.huffingtonpost.com/jeffrey-bland/chronic-illness-what-work_b_281228.html

Brocker, C., Thompson, D. C., & Vasiliou, V. (2012). The role of hyperosmotic stress in inflammation and disease. *Biomolecular Concepts*, *3*(4), 345-364.

Center for Disease Control. (2012). NCHS Data Brief, 75 Years of Mortality in the United States, 1935–2010.

Chin Lye, C., Jones, M., & Kingham, J. C. (2007). Celiac Disease and Autoimmune Thyroid Disease. *Clinical Medicine & Research*, *5*(3), 184-192.

Ciarrocca, M., Tomei, F., Caciari, T., Cetica, C., Andr, J., Fiaschetti, M., & ... Sancini, A. (2012). Exposure to Arsenic in urban and rural areas and effects on thyroid hormones. *Inhalation Toxicology*, *24*(9), 589-598.

de Souza da Fonseca, A., Mencalha, A., Araújo de Campos, V., Ferreira Machado, S., de Freitas Peregrino, A., Geller, M., &

de Paoli, F. (2013). DNA repair gene expression in biological tissues exposed to low-intensity infrared laser. *Lasers in Medical Science*, *28*(4), 1077-1084.

E. Niedermeyer, F. Lopes Da Silva (Eds.), EEG: Basic Principles, Clinical and Related Fields, Williams & Wilkins, Baltimore, MD (1993), pp. 581–596.

Elkan, A., Sjöberg, B., Kolsrud, B., Ringertz, B., Hafström, I., & Frostegård, J. (2008). Gluten-free vegan diet induces decreased LDL and oxidized LDL levels and raised atheroprotective natural antibodies against phosphorylcholine in patients with rheumatoid arthritis: a randomized study. *Arthritis Research & Therapy*, *10*(2), R34.

Farhat, S. L., Silva, C. A., Orione, M. M., Campos, L. A., Sallum, A. E., & Braga, A. F. (2011). Air pollution in autoimmune rheumatic diseases: A review. *Autoimmunity Reviews*,*11*(1), 14-21.

Fleming, L., Kirkpatrick, B., Backer, L., Bean, J., Wanner, A., Dalpra, D., & ... Baden, D. (2005). Initial evaluation of the effects of aerosolized Florida red tide toxins (brevetoxins) in persons with asthma. *Environmental Health Perspectives*, *113*(5), 650-657.

Frech, H.E., Parente, S.T., & Hoff, J. (2012). US Health Care: A Reality Check on Cross-Country Comparisons. *American Enterprise Institute.*

Growing Number of Autoimmune Disease Cases Reported. (2012, June 21).American Autoimmune Related Diseases Association (AARDA). Retrieved from http://www.newswise.com/articles/growing-number-of-autoimmune-disease-cases-reported

Hadjivassiliou, M. M., Grünewald, R. A., Kandler, R. H., Chattopadhyay, A. K., Jarratt, J. A., Sanders, D. S., & ... Davies-Jones, G. B. (2006).

Neuropathy associated with gluten sensitivity. *Journal of Neurology, Neurosurgery & Psychiatry*, *77*(11), 1262-1266.

Hadjivassiliou, M., Sanders, D., Grünewald, R., Woodroofe, N., Boscolo, S., & Aeschlimann, D. (2010). Gluten sensitivity: from gut to brain. *Lancet Neurology*, *9*(3), 318-330.

Heck, J., Chen, Y., Grann, V., Slavkovich, V., Parvez, F., & Ahsan, H. (2008). Arsenic exposure and anemia in Bangladesh: a population-based study. *Journal of Occupational & Environmental Medicine*, *50*(1), 80-87.

Holloway, J. W., Savarimuthu Francis, S., Fong, K. M., & Yang, I. A. (2012). Genomics and the respiratory effects of air pollution exposure. *Respirology*, *17*(4), 590-600.

Hong, S., Weng-Im, L., Jian-Qing, R., Song-Lin, L., Pui-Cheong Lei, J., Yi-Tao, W., & Ru, Y. (2013). Biotransformation of ginsenoside Rb1 via the gypenoside pathway by human gut bacteria. *Chinese Medicine*, *8*(1), 22-33.

Krajmalnik-Brown, R., Ilhan, Z., Kang, D., & DiBaise, J. K. (2012). Effects of Gut Microbes on Nutrient Absorption and Energy Regulation. *Nutrition In Clinical Practice*, *27*(2), 201-214.

Kurd, B., Dar, M., Shoaib, M., Malik, L., Aijaz, Z., & Asif, I. (2014). Relationship between stress and coronary heart disease. *Asian Cardiovascular & Thoracic Annals*, *22*(2), 142-147.

Lichtwark, I. T., Newnham, E. D., Robinson, S. R., Shepherd, S. J., Hosking, P. P., Gibson, P. R., & Yelland, G. W. (2014). Cognitive impairment in coeliac disease improves on a gluten-free diet and correlates with histological and serological indices of disease severity. *Alimentary Pharmacology & Therapeutics*, *40*(2), 160-170.

Mahapatra, L. (2013, January 17). CHART OF THE DAY: Americans Will Continue To Spend More On Drugs Than The Rest Of The World In 2016. Business Insider. Retrieved from http://www.businessinsider.com/us-spending-more-on-pharmaceuticals-2013-1#ixzz35E3MtpWt

Martin, G. (1999, August 2). Our Poisoned Bay / Despite end to direct piping of sewage, pollution worse now than 30 years ago. SFGate. Retrieved from http://www.sfgate.com/news/article/Our-Poisoned-Bay-Despite-end-to-direct-piping-2914964.php

Meyers, B. A. (2013). PEMF-*The Fifth Element* of *Health: Learn Why Pulsed Electromagnetic Field Therapy (PEMF) Supercharges Your Health Like Nothing Else*. Bloomington, Ind.: Balboa Press.

Morris, T., Moore, M., & Morris, F. (2011). Stress and Chronic Illness: the Case of Diabetes. *Journal of Adult Development*, *18*(2), 70-80.

O'Toole, T., Conklin, D., & Bhatnagar, A. (2008). Environmental risk factors for heart disease. Reviews On Environmental Health, 23(3), 167-202.

Paolo, W. (2014). *The "Standard of Care"*. Emergency Medicine at SUNY Upstate.

Perlmutter, D. (2010, November 2). Neurogenesis: How to Change Your Brain. The Huffington Post. Retrieved from http://www.huffingtonpost.com/dr-david-perlmutter-md/neurogenesis-what-it-mean_b_777163.html

Ritz, S. (2010). Air pollution as a potential contributor to the 'epidemic' of autoimmune disease. *Medical Hypotheses*, *74*(1), 110-117.

Robinson, S., Leach, J., Owen-Lynch, P., & Sünram-Lea, S. (2013). Stress reactivity and cognitive performance in a simulated firefighting emergency. *Aviation, Space, And Environmental Medicine*, *84*(6), 592-599.

Rodrigues, N. C., Assis, L., Fernandes, K. R., Magri, A., Ribeiro, D. A., Brunelli, R., & ... Renno, A. M. (2013). Effects of 660 nm low-level laser therapy on muscle healing process after cryolesion. *Journal Of Rehabilitation Research & Development*, *50*(7), 985-995.

Santos, S., Alves, A., Leal-Junior, E., Albertini, R., Vieira, R., Ligeiro, A., & ... Carvalho, P. (2014). Comparative analysis of two low-level laser doses on the expression of inflammatory mediators and on neutrophils and macrophages in acute joint inflammation. *Lasers in Medical Science*, *29*(3), 1051-1058.

Shetty, S., Marathe, N., Lanjekar, V., Ranade, D., & Shouche, Y. S. (2013). Comparative Genome Analysis of Megasphaera sp. Reveals Niche Specialization and Its Potential Role in the Human Gut. *Plos ONE*, *8*(11), 1-13.

VanEngelenburg, G. (2013). Low-Level Laser Acupuncture and the Use of the Respond Luminex Vet Class 3b Laser. *American Journal Of Traditional Chinese Veterinary Medicine*, *8*(2), 73-76.

Wilson, G. S., & George, J. (2014). Physical and chemical insults induce inflammation and gastrointestinal cancers. *Cancer Letters*, *345*(2), 190-195.